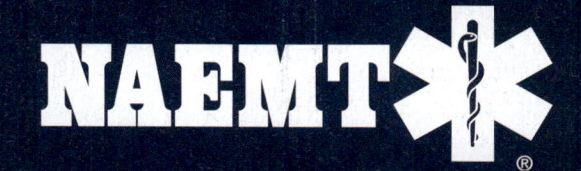

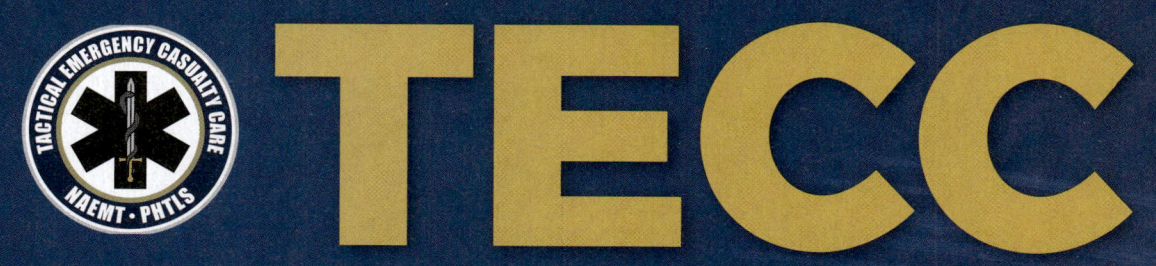

TECC
Tactical Emergency Casualty Care
SECOND EDITION

Course Manual

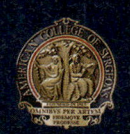

Endorsed By American College of Surgeons COMMITTEE ON TRAUMA

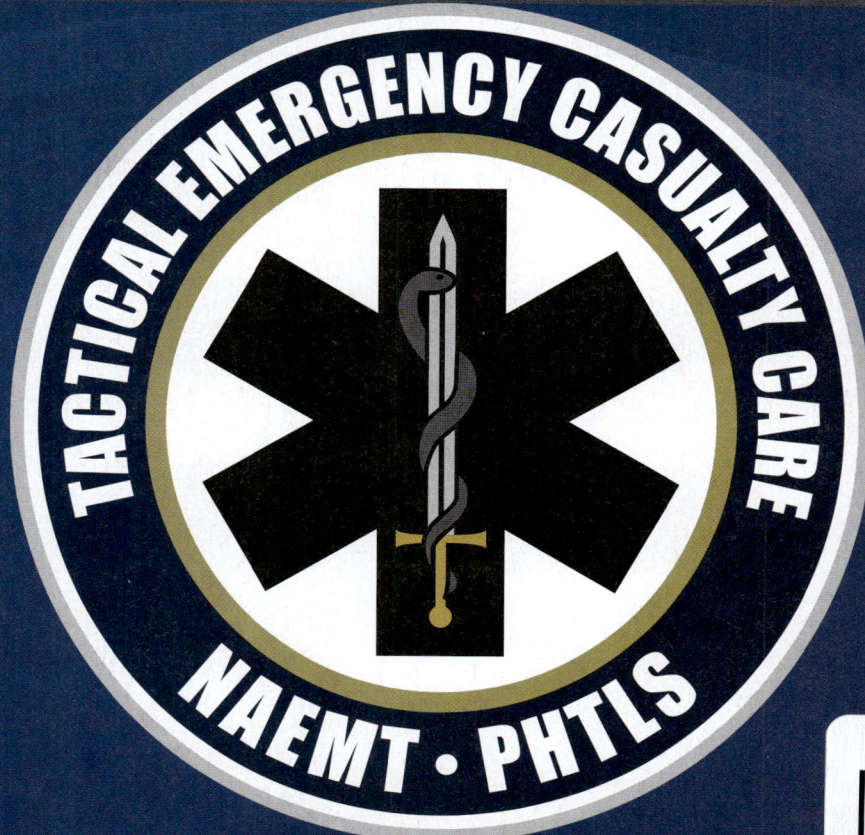

Recognized Program Of

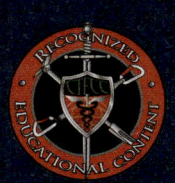

TECC

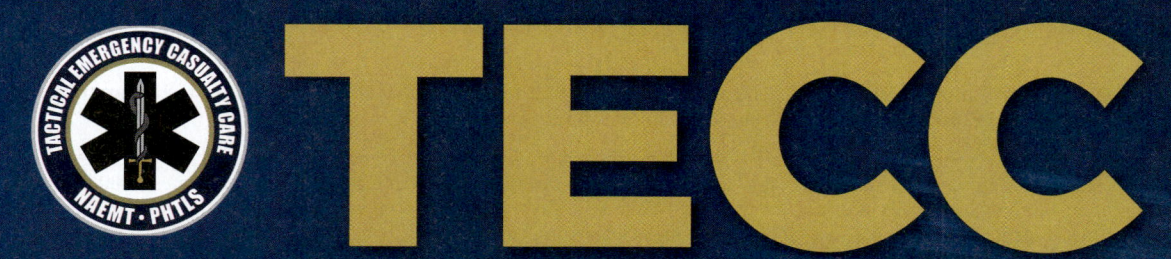

Tactical Emergency Casualty Care

SECOND EDITION

Course Manual

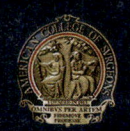

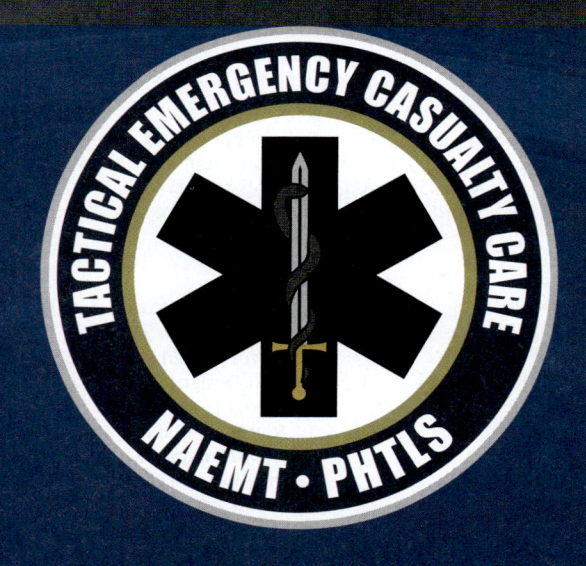

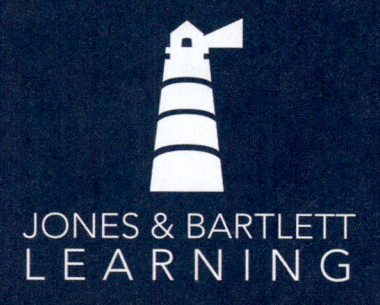

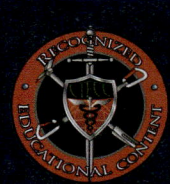

NAEMT

Endorsed By American College of Surgeons COMMITTEE ON TRAUMA

JONES & BARTLETT LEARNING

Recognized Program Of

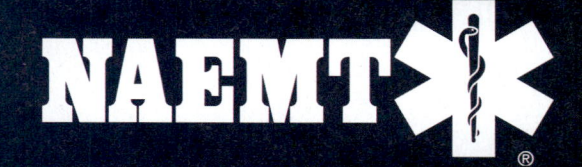

World Headquarters
Jones & Bartlett Learning
25 Mall Road
Burlington, MA 01803
978-443-5000
info@jblearning.com
www.jblearning.com

Jones & Bartlett Learning books and products are available through most bookstores and online booksellers. To contact Jones & Bartlett Learning directly, call 800-832-0034, fax 978-443-8000, or visit our website, www.jblearning.com.

> Substantial discounts on bulk quantities of Jones & Bartlett Learning publications are available to corporations, professional associations, and other qualified organizations. For details and specific discount information, contact the special sales department at Jones & Bartlett Learning via the above contact information or send an email to specialsales@jblearning.com.

Copyright © 2020 by National Association of Emergency Medical Technicians (NAEMT)

All rights reserved. No part of the material protected by this copyright may be reproduced or utilized in any form, electronic or mechanical, including photocopying, recording, or by any information storage and retrieval system, without written permission from the copyright owner.

The content, statements, views, and opinions herein are the sole expression of the respective authors and not that of Jones & Bartlett Learning, LLC. Reference herein to any specific commercial product, process, or service by trade name, trademark, manufacturer, or otherwise does not constitute or imply its endorsement or recommendation by Jones & Bartlett Learning, LLC and such reference shall not be used for advertising or product endorsement purposes. All trademarks displayed are the trademarks of the parties noted herein. *Tactical Emergency Casualty Care Course Manual, Second Edition* is an independent publication and has not been authorized, sponsored, or otherwise approved by the owners of the trademarks or service marks referenced in this product.

There may be images in this book that feature models; these models do not necessarily endorse, represent, or participate in the activities represented in the images. Any screenshots in this product are for educational and instructive purposes only. Any individuals and scenarios featured in the case studies throughout this product may be real or fictitious, but are used for instructional purposes only.

The procedures and protocols in this book are based on the most current recommendations of responsible medical sources. The National Association of Emergency Medical Technicians (NAEMT) and the publisher, however, make no guarantee as to, and assume no responsibility for, the correctness, sufficiency, or completeness of such information or recommendations. Other or additional safety measures may be required under particular circumstances.

This textbook is intended solely as a guide to the appropriate procedures to be employed when rendering emergency care to the sick and injured. It is not intended as a statement of the standards of care required in any particular situation, because circumstances and the patient's physical condition can vary widely from one emergency to another. Nor is it intended that this textbook shall in any way advise emergency personnel concerning legal authority to perform the activities or procedures discussed. Such local determination should be made only with the aid of legal counsel.

21403-1

Production Credits
General Manager and Executive Publisher: Kimberly Brophy
VP, Product Development: Christine Emerton
Senior Managing Editor: Donna Gridley
Product Manager: Tiffany Sliter
Senior Content Developer: Jennifer Deforge-Kling
VP, Sales, Public Safety Group: Matthew Maniscalco
Project Specialist: Nora Menzi
Digital Products Manager: Jordan McKenzie
Director of Marketing Operations: Brian Rooney
Production Services Manager: Colleen Lamy
VP, Manufacturing and Inventory Control: Therese Connell
Composition: S4Carlisle Publishing Services
Cover Design: Kristin E. Parker
Text Design: Kristin E. Parker
Media Development Editor: Troy Liston
Rights & Media Specialist: Rebecca Damon
Cover Image: © Ralf Hiemisch/Getty Images
Printing and Binding: LSC Communications
Cover Printing: LSC Communications

Library of Congress Cataloging-in-Publication Data
Names: National Association of Emergency Medical Technicians (U.S.), issuing body.
Title: Tactical emergency casualty care (TECC) : course manual / National Association of Emergency Medical Technicians.
Other titles: TECC
Description: Second edition. | Burlington, MA : Jones & Bartlett Learning, [2020] | Includes bibliographical references and index.
Identifiers: LCCN 2019008226 | ISBN 9781284483871 (pbk.)
Subjects: | MESH: Emergency Treatment | Wounds, Gunshot--therapy | Emergency Medical Technicians | Mass Casualty Incidents--prevention & control | Civil Defense | Guideline
Classification: LCC RD96.3 | NLM WO 807 | DDC 617.1/45--dc23
LC record available at https://lccn.loc.gov/2019008226

6048

Printed in the United States of America
26 25 24 23 22   10 9 8 7 6 5 4

Brief Contents

Lesson 1 Introduction to Tactical Emergency Combat Care...................................1

Lesson 2 Direct Threat Care/Hot Zone............7

Lesson 3 Indirect Threat Care/Warm Zone: MARCH—Patient Assessment and Massive Hemorrhage Interventions.......................17

Lesson 4 Indirect Threat Care/Warm Zone: MARCH—Airway...................................27

Lesson 5 Indirect Threat Care/Warm Zone: Respiration/Breathing 41

Lesson 6 Indirect Threat Care/Warm Zone: MARCH—Circulation........................53

Lesson 7 Indirect Threat Care/Warm Zone: Hypothermia and Head Injury 69

Lesson 8 Evacuation Care/Cold Zone 83

Lesson 9 Triage 99

Lesson 10 Summation 107

Table of Contents

Lesson 1 Introduction to Tactical Emergency Combat Care 1

Introduction to Tactical Emergency Casualty Care 1
- Where Did the Tactical Emergency Casualty Care Course Come From? 1

What Does the Tactical Emergency Casualty Care Course Cover? 2

Tactical Care Situations 3
- Resuscitation Zones: Phases of Care 3

NAEMT TECC Course Goals 4
- TECC Guiding Principles 4
- Response and Arrival-Scene Assessment 5

Other Elements Operating Within a Tactical Environment 5
- Rescue Task Force 5
- Tactical Emergency Medical Support 6

Summary 6
References and Resources 6

Lesson 2 Direct Threat Care/Hot Zone 7

Direct Threat Care/Hot Zone 7
- Operating in the Direct Threat Care/Hot Zone 7
- Get Off the X 7
- Constantly Changing Threat Environment 7
- Cover Versus Concealment 8
- Mitigation of Direct Threats 8

Rescue Considerations 8
- Rapid and Remote Assessment Methodology 8
- Operational Performance 10
- Drag and Carry Options 10

Medical Interventions in the Direct Threat Care/Hot Zone 12
- Place Patient in the Recovery Position 12
- Controlling Massive Hemorrhage 12
- Types of Tourniquets 13

Summary 14
Skill Stations 14
- Casualty Drags and Carries 14
- Tourniquet Application 15

References and Resources 15

Lesson 3 Indirect Threat Care/Warm Zone: MARCH—Patient Assessment and Massive Hemorrhage Interventions 17

Indirect Threat Care/Warm Zone 17
- Scene Safety 17
- Asymmetrical Response 18
- Threat Management 18

Assessment and Intervention Priorities 18
- Bleeding Assessment 19

Progressive and Aggressive Intervention Plan ... 20
- Direct Pressure 20

Extremity Tourniquets 21
- Tourniquet Optimization 21
- Venous Tourniquets 22
- Tourniquet Conversion Contradictions 22

Junctional Hemorrhage 22
- Junctional Tourniquets 22
- The Combat Ready Clamp 22
- The Junctional Emergency Treatment Tool 23
- The SAM Junctional Tourniquet 23

Hemostatic Dressings 23
- Combat Gauze Directions 24

Summary 24
Skill Stations 24
- Inguinal Hemorrhage 24
- Axillary Hemorrhage 25

References 25

Lesson 4 Indirect Threat Care/Warm Zone: MARCH—Airway 27

Overview of Airway in the Indirect Threat Care/Warm Zone 27
- Trauma Jaw Thrust and Chin Lift Maneuvers 27
- Nasopharyngeal Airway 28
- Recovery Position 29
- The Sit-Up/Lean Forward Position 29

Complex Airways 29
- Supraglottic Airways 29
- Orotracheal and Nasotracheal Intubation 31

Surgical Cricothyrotomy 31
- Cricothyrotomy Surface Landmarks 32
- Cricothyrotomy Incision 33
- Insert and Secure Endotracheal Tube 34

Table of Contents vii

 Bougie-Assisted Placement of ET Tube
  in Surgical Airway 35
Pediatric Airways **36**
 Pediatric Nasopharyngeal Airway 36
 Pediatric Supraglottic Airway 37
 Advanced Pediatric Airways 38
Summary **39**
Skill Sheets **39**
 Nasopharyngeal Airway 39
 Supraglottic Airway 39
 Emergency Surgical Airway 39
References **40**

Lesson 5 Indirect Threat Care/Warm Zone: Respiration/Breathing 41

Overview of Respiration/Breathing
 Indirect Threat Care/Warm Zone **41**
 Anatomy and Physiology of Breathing 41
 The Oxygenation and Ventilation Process 43
 Pathophysiology 43
Open Pneumothorax **44**
 Assessment and Management of an Open
  Pneumothorax 44
Chest Seals **46**
Tension Pneumothorax **47**
 Assessment and Management of a Tension
  Pneumothorax 47
Needle Decompression **48**
 TECC Needle Decompression Procedure 49
 Assessing the Effectiveness of Needle
  Decompression 50
 Bilateral Needle Decompression for
  Traumatic Cardiac Arrest 50
 Pediatric Tension Pneumothorax 50
Summary **50**
Skill Station **50**
 Needle Decompression 50
References and Resources **51**

Lesson 6 Indirect Threat Care/Warm Care: MARCH—Circulation 53

Overview of Circulation Indirect Threat
 Care/Warm Zone **53**
 Tourniquet Assessment and Application in
  Indirect Threat Care/Warm Zone 53
 Tourniquet Application 54
 Application Tightness 55
 Time Limit 55
Pelvic Binders **55**
 Stabilization of Pelvic Fractures 56
 Control of Pelvic Hemorrhage 56
 Indications and Contradictions for Pelvic
  Binder Use 56
 Application of Pelvic Binder 56

Shock Assessment **56**
Hypovolemic Shock **58**
Hemorrhagic Shock **58**
Fluid Resuscitation of Hemorrhagic Shock **60**
Neurogenic Shock **61**
Intravenous Access **62**
 Intraosseous Access 62
Tranexamic Acid **64**
 TXA Administration 65
Damage Control Resuscitation **65**
 Coagulopathy and the "Lethal Triad" 65
 TECC Damage Control Resuscitation 66
Traumatic Brain Injury **66**
Summary **66**
Skill Stations **66**
 Intraosseous Access 67
 IV Administration of TXA 67
References **68**

Lesson 7 Indirect Threat Care/Warm Zone: Hypothermia and Head Injury 69

Overview of Circulation Indirect
 Threat Care/Warm Zone **69**
Hypothermia **69**
 Hypothermia Aspect of the Lethal Triad 70
 Preventing Hypothermia 70
 Hypothermia Prevention and Management Kits 71
Traumatic Brain Injury Assessment and
 Intervention **71**
 Glasgow Coma Scale 71
 Cushing's Triad 72
 Intracranial Hypertension 72
 TBI Intervention 72
Reassess, Monitor, and Document Patient **72**
 Secondary Survey 73
 Obtaining Vital Signs 74
 Monitoring 74
 Documentation 74
Analgesia **75**
 Ketamine 75
Fire and Bombs as Weapons **75**
 Public Safety Fire Ignition Sources 76
 Explosives 76
Burn Care **76**
 Assessment of Burn Injury 77
 Fluid Resuscitation of Burned Patients 78
 Smoke Inhalation: Fluid Management
  Considerations 78
 Analgesia 79
Penetrating Eye Trauma **79**
 Care for Penetrating Eye Trauma 79
Moving and Communicating With
 the Patient **79**

Communicating With the Patient....................79
Communicating With Receiving Hospitals..........80
CPR in a Multicasualty Event 80
Correct Tension Pneumothorax....................80
Summary..80
References.. 81

Lesson 8 Evacuation Care/Cold Zone......................83

Overview of Evacuation Care/Cold Zone.........83
Differences Between Indirect Threat Care/Warm Zone and Evacuation Care/Cold Zone 83
Situational Awareness in Evacuation Care/Cold Zone..83
Have Primary, Secondary, and Tertiary Evacuation Plans...............................84
Evacuation Care Transport Resources...............84
Evacuation Care: Reassessment 85
Airway..85
Supraglottic Airways..............................85
Breathing...86
Needle Decompression............................86
Evacuation Care: Hemorrhage Control 87
Tranexamic Acid 87
Tourniquet Assessment and Conversion.........88
Tourniquet Conversion Procedures................88
Plus-1 Tourniquet.................................88
Contraindications for Tourniquet Conversion.........90
Evacuation Care: Shock Management...........90
Establish IV or Intraosseous (IO) line..............90
Evacuation Care: Traumatic Brain Injury........90
Altered Mental Status With Suspected TBI........... 91
Fluid Resuscitation of TBI 91
Evacuation Care: Burns 91
CYANOKIT 92
Amyl Nitrite......................................92
Sodium Thiosulfate 92
Example of a Hydrogen Cyanide Poisoning Protocol......................92
Evacuation Care: Analgesia......................93
Evacuation Care: CPR...........................93
Evacuation Care: Hypothermia 95
Evacuation Care: Reassess, Document, Communicate, and Prepare for Movement....95
Communicating With the Patient..................95
Communicating With Receiving Hospitals...........96
Preparing for Patient Movement...................96
Summary..96
References and Resources.......................96

Lesson 9 Triage.......................99

Overview of TECC Triage........................99
Triage Concepts 99
Primary Triage..................................100
Limitations of Triage Systems 100
START Triage................................... 101
SALT Triage 101
Sacco Triage Method...........................103
Secondary Triage Decisions.....................103
Tactical Situation................................103
Casualty Response to MARCH Treatments..........104
Summary..104
REFERENCES...................................105

Lesson 10 Summation 107

Overview of Summation Lesson 107
Importance of Immediate Responders.........107
Phases of TECC Care 108
Direct Threat Care/Hot Zone 108
Indirect Threat Care/Warm Zone..................108
Evacuation Care/Cold Zone 108
Direct Threat Care/Hot Zone Goals 109
Rapid and Remote Assessment Methodology......109
Stop the Bleeding................................109
Drags and Carries................................109
Indirect Threat Care/Warm Zone Goals......... 110
Indirect Threat/Warm Zone Triage 110
Indirect Threat Care/Warm Zone: Bleeding Control............................... 111
Indirect Threat Care/Warm Zone: Airway Control................................. 111
Recovery Position 112
Cricothyrotomy 112
Tension Pneumothorax.........................112
Open Pneumothorax 113
Indirect Threat Care/Warm Zone: Shock Control..................................114
Indirect Threat Care/Warm Zone: Analgesics....114
Evacuation Care 115
Summary..115
Reference.......................................115

Index 131

Acknowledgments

We would like to thank all NAEMT tactical faculty on behalf of the National Association of Emergency Medical Technicians (NAEMT) for their contributions as members of NAEMT's tactical faculty. Whether currently serving as a Tactical Emergency Casualty Care (TECC) instructor, a Tactical Combat Casualty Care (TCCC) instructor, or both, your service as a member of our faculty is a key factor in the great success of our programs. You are responsible for providing prehospital providers with the knowledge and skills they need to make the best decisions in the field for their patients. Thank you for what you do each and every day for your students and communities.

To all NAEMT tactical students, thank you for the courageous work you do in the field each and every day. We hope that this NAEMT TECC course provides you with the knowledge and skills you need to make the best decisions in the field for your patients, in the event of an active shooter or other hostile event.

NAEMT is committed to field testing all new and revised courses before release to the public. The second edition of the TECC course was field tested on four occasions, and we would like to thank all involved.

In addition to the core author team, we would like to thank the instructors who helped teach in Las Vegas—Phil Carey, John Phelps, Lee Richardson, Bob Waddell, and Ron Wenzel; and at Tinker Air Force Base in Oklahoma—Chad Beals. For teaching the TECC beta materials to hundreds of prehospital providers in Hawaii, we would like to thank Barbara Brennan, Dr. Elizabeth Char, Mike Jones, David Kingdon, and Jeff Zuckernick. And finally, through the Indiana Department of Homeland Security, teaching in Greenwood, Indiana, thank you to Mike Brown and Mark Litwinko.

TECC Course Author Team

Alexander L. Eastman, MD, MPH, FACS, FAEMS*
Senior Medical Officer, U.S. Department of Homeland Security
Countering Weapons of Mass Destruction Office
Lieutenant and Chief Medical Officer, Dallas Police Department
Dallas, Texas

David Flory, BS, Paramedic
Lead Instructor, VALOR Officer Safety and Wellness Program
Institute for Intergovernmental Research
Chief of Police, Retired
Hot Springs, Arkansas

Donald C. Heath, Jr., BS, NR-P, TP-C
Master Deputy Sheriff/Paramedic
Special Weapons and Tactics (SWAT)/Aviation
Lake County Sheriff's Office
Tavares, Florida

Michael J. Hunter, NREMTP
Deputy Chief EMS
Worcester EMS at UMass Memorial Medical Center, University Campus
Member, Massachusetts State Police STOP Team Medical Support Group
Worcester, Massachusetts

William (Bill) Justice, NRP, TEMS-I
Associate Director
Center for Prehospital and Disaster Medicine
University of Oklahoma Department of Emergency Medicine
U.S. Marshals Task Force
Oklahoma Highway Patrol Special Operations
Oklahoma County Sheriffs Tactical Team
Tulsa, Oklahoma

Richard A. Nydam, Paramedic
Training and Education Specialist
Worcester EMS at UMass Memorial Medical Center, University Campus
Member, Massachusetts State Police STOP Team Medical Support Group
Adjunct Faculty and Clinical Coordinator
Quinsigamond Community College Paramedic Program
Worcester, Massachusetts

Julie Chase, MSEd, FAWM, TP-C
Tactical Medicine Instructor
Instructional Systems Designer
U.S. Department of State
Berryville, Virginia

---

*The work of the authors does not represent an official publication of the United States Government or the Department of Homeland Security.

Contributors

TECC Course Contributors

Michael Costanza
Brendan Hartford, EMT-P, NRP
Mike Meoli, TP-C
Geoff Shapiro, MD
Reed Smith, MD
The Fisdap Team

LESSON 1

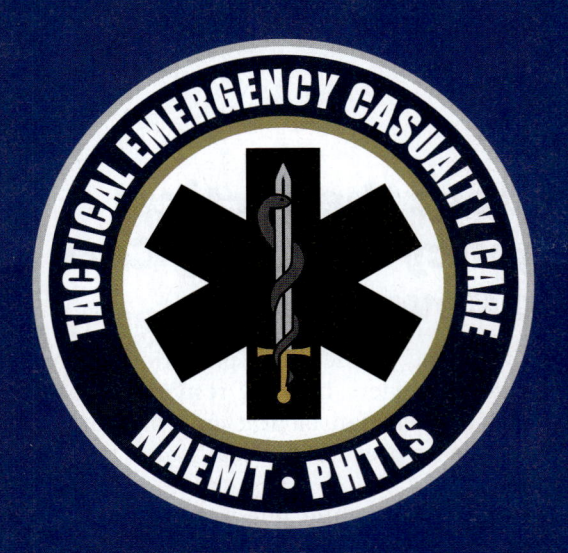

Introduction to Tactical Emergency Casualty Care

LESSON OBJECTIVES
- Describe the key factors influencing casualty care.
- Discuss the impacts that threat, time, incident, location, and available resources have on the tactical response and care of trauma patients.
- Understand how Tactical Combat Casualty Care (TCCC) and Tactical Emergency Casualty Care (TECC) were developed.
- Describe the phases of tactical casualty care.
- Explain the differences between military tactical and civilian tactical prehospital trauma care.

Introduction to Tactical Emergency Casualty Care

TECC is a set of best practice treatment guidelines for trauma care in the high-threat prehospital environment. These guidelines are built upon critical medical lessons learned by U.S. and allied military forces during 21st-century conflict and brought to the civilian sector via the Committee on Tactical Combat Casualty Care (Co-TCCC). They are appropriately modified to address the specific needs of civilian populations and civilian emergency medical services (EMS) practice. The guidelines are freely available to all interested stakeholders.

Response to mass-casualty events, such as the shootings at the Route 91 Harvest country music festival in Las Vegas and the bombings at the 2013 Boston Marathon, demonstrated the gap that exists between the capability of prehospital trauma care and casualty needs during these events. In fact, the Federal Emergency Management Agency (FEMA) has identified mass-casualty incident (MCI) preparation as a national priority. The National Association of Emergency Medical Technicians (NAEMT) second edition TECC course is designed to provide caregivers with best practices when operating in a high-risk environment involving multiple casualties (**Figure 1-1**).

Where Did the Tactical Emergency Casualty Care Course Come From?

This TECC course was developed using guidelines from the Committee for Tactical Emergency Casualty Care (C-TECC). Formed in 2010, the C-TECC formally translated military trauma lessons into the civilian

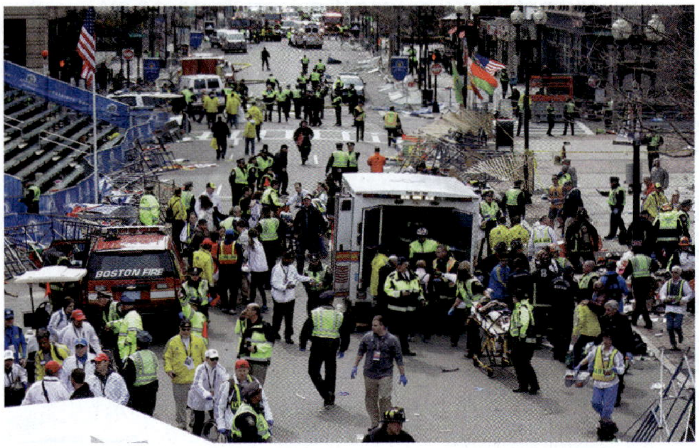

Figure 1-1 Mass-casualty management at the scene of the Boston Marathon bombing.
© Charles Krupa/AP Images.

high-threat prehospital community. The committee brought together subject matter experts from EMS, fire, law enforcement, and the Department of Homeland Security to work with physicians from emergency departments, trauma centers, and the military to develop best practices for high-threat prehospital medicine.

The C-TECC is modeled after the highly successful U.S. Department of Defense Co-TCCC—frequently credited as one of the major initiatives that has resulted in the lowest combat mortality rates in recorded history. However, Co-TCCC treatment guidelines focus on a very specific population: fit and healthy 18- to 40-year olds in a combat environment.

The C-TECC guidelines, therefore, cover the requirements of a civilian population. This includes pediatric, geriatric, and special needs patients, as well as considerations for underlying medical conditions common in a civilian population, the characteristics and limitations of civilian EMS, and the varied types of threats that responders face. TECC guidelines have since been incorporated into the National Joint Counterterrorism Awareness Workshop used by the FBI, FEMA, and the National Counterterrorism Center. The NAEMT TECC course is built from four information sources:

- U.S. Department of Defense Tactical Combat Casualty Care (TCCC) course
- Committee for Tactical Emergency Casualty Care (C-TECC) guidelines
- Prehospital Trauma Committee of NAEMT
- National Tactical Emergency Medical Support (TEMS) competency domains

The NAEMT TECC course focuses on prehospital medical care in high-risk tactical situations. TECC is not a comprehensive tactical operators' course. Completing TECC does not result in certification as a tactical medic. In addition, the TECC course is not a rescue task force course.

CHECK YOUR KNOWLEDGE

TECC guidelines cover the medical requirements of:

a. fit and healthy 18- to 40-year-old first responders.
b. emergency medical services responders.
c. those most likely to survive a multisystem trauma injury.
d. the civilian population.

What Does the Tactical Emergency Casualty Care Course Cover?

NAEMT's TECC course teaches EMS practitioners and other prehospital providers how to respond to and care for patients in a civilian tactical environment. It is designed to decrease preventable deaths in a tactical situation.

The course presents the three phases of tactical care:

- Direct threat care that is rendered while under attack or in adverse conditions.
- Indirect threat care that is rendered while the threat has been suppressed but may resurface at any point.
- Evacuation care that is rendered while the casualty is being evacuated from the incident site.

The 16-hour classroom course covers the following topics:

- Hemorrhage control
- Surgical airway control and needle decompression
- Strategies for treating wounded responders in threatening environments
- Caring for pediatric patients
- Techniques for dragging and carrying victims to safety

The course includes EMT, advanced EMT, and paramedic skills. It is NAEMT's philosophy that TECC caregivers should be exposed to all skills in this course. As such, students may practice a skill in the TECC class that is beyond their current scope of practice. The value of this exposure is that the TECC caregiver can anticipate what procedures will be done in an actual tactical situation and the time required to complete the skill. Students are expected to participate in all in-class skills required in a TECC course. Outside of class, all clinical interventions must be in accordance with local policy and protocol and within the caregiver's authorized scope of practice.

The TECC course offers the following skill stations:

- Casualty drags, carries, and assists
- Tourniquets
- Tourniquet optimization
- Junctional tourniquets
- Wound packing/compression dressing
- Airway management
- Chest seals/needle decompression (NDC)

- MARCH assessment/shock assessment
- Intravenous (IV)/intraosseous (IO) fluid administration

> **CHECK YOUR KNOWLEDGE**
>
> You have successfully completed the TECC course and are operating in an indirect threat care/warm zone scene. Your patient has a tension pneumothorax, is rapidly decompensating, and needs a needle decompression. You can perform this skill under which of these situations?
>
> a. On-site medical oversight is available by a critical care paramedic or physician assistant.
> b. The caregiver calls medical control, identifies as a TECC-credentialed caregiver, and obtains authorization.
> c. Needle decompression is within the caregiver's scope of practice and authorized under local policy and protocol.
> d. The incident has been declared a mass-casualty event and the authority having jurisdiction has established medical incident command under the National Response Framework.

Tactical Care Situations

Active shooter/hostile events (ASHEs) have been increasing in severity and frequency since 2000. The distribution of such events has impacted rural, suburban, and urban communities. What makes these events unique from other mass-casualty events is that responders are at high risk for injury or death when arriving at an ASHE incident. In addition, the use of military-style weapons and techniques results in patients with complex and life-threatening traumatic wounds.

Resuscitation Zones: Phases of Care

TECC divides patient care into three zones that match the disaster management and EMS identification of caregiver and patient risk. Each zone has specific treatment goals, caregiver skills, and patient management objectives. Casualty scenarios in dynamic events usually entail both a medical problem and a tactical problem. The TECC goal is: Right Care—Right Time—Right Patient.

Direct Threat Care/Hot Zone

This zone (or phase) represents the highest danger to caregiver and patient. There is an immediate threat of additional injury or death. The incident scene is not secure. The emphasis in this zone is on threat suppression, preventing further casualties, extracting casualties from the high-threat area, and implementing control of life-threatening hemorrhage.

Indirect Threat Care/Warm Zone

Later lessons will extensively cover TECC operations in the indirect threat care/warm zone. The warm zone is the area where a potential threat exists, but there is no direct or immediate threat. For example, if you are called to an active shooter situation at a local mall, you may need to enter the mall to tend to casualties. Wherever the shooter is contained, but still active, is considered the hot zone (direct threat care). The rest of the mall would be the warm zone, as the shooter could escape containment and become an immediate threat in your area. Warm zone care includes the other lifesaving interventions associated with applying the MARCH algorithm (**M**assive hemorrhage, **A**irway, **R**espiration, **C**irculation, and **H**ead/Hypothermia). Casualty collection points and rescue task forces are typically employed within the warm zone.

Evacuation Care/Cold Zone

Evacuation care/cold zone is the area where no significant threat is reasonably anticipated, and additional medical/transport resources may be staged. Evacuation care generally falls under established local, regional, or state protocols (**Figure 1-2**).

Table 1-1 provides examples of the different zones and phases of care.

> **CHECK YOUR KNOWLEDGE**
>
> The use of advanced airway devices can start in the _____ zone.
>
> a. direct threat/hot
> b. indirect threat/warm
> c. evacuation/cold
> d. All of the zones

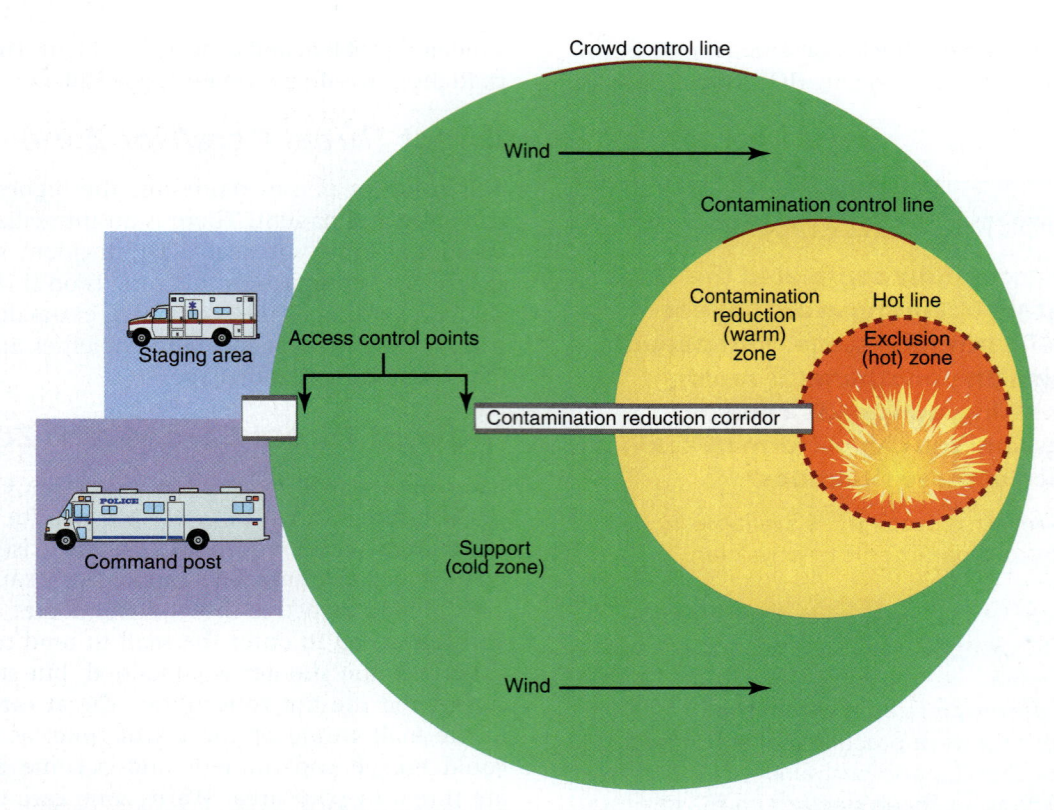

Figure 1-2 Direct threat, indirect threat, and evacuation care are matched with the hot zone, warm zone, and cold zone descriptions used by emergency management.
© National Association of Emergency Medical Technicians (NAEMT).

Table 1-1 Zones and Phases of Care

Zone/Phase of Care	Examples
Direct threat/hot zone	■ You are in the direct line of fire of an active shooter. ■ Someone is deploying a biologic weapon and you are in the contamination zone.
Indirect threat/warm zone	■ There is an active shooter in the area, but you are not in the line of fire.
Evacuation/cold zone	■ You are transporting casualties to the hospital from the scene of an ASHE.

NAEMT TECC Course Goals

The NAEMT course goals for TECC are designed to provide the caregiver with evidence-based best practices when responding to an ASHE with many patients:

- Rapid assessment of the trauma patient
- Student knowledge regarding examination and diagnostic skills
- Understanding the three phases of care
- Enhancing student assessment and treatment of the trauma patient
- Advancing student competence in prehospital trauma intervention skills in tactical environments
- Establishing management of the multisystem trauma patient while limiting the risk of further casualties
- Promoting a common approach for the initiation and transition of care of the trauma patient
- Providing an understanding of tactical and environmental factors on trauma care

TECC Guiding Principles

Responding to and working within an ASHE tactical situation requires a different response from EMS caregivers. C-TECC guidelines provide four guiding principles for caregivers:

Casualty Scenarios in Dynamic Events Usually Entail Both a Medical Problem and a Tactical Problem

Not all tactical events will be initially dispatched as an ASHE. It may start as a request for an ambulance for a "person down in the street." A "sudden impact" mass-casualty event is one that causes traumatic injuries involving burns, fractures, bleeding, and trauma as well as death. A conventional mass-casualty event does not contain any chemical, biologic, radiologic, or nuclear (CBRN) elements.

An "emergency" mass-casualty event describes an event that generates hundreds of casualties, occurs simultaneously in multiple locations, or involves CBRN elements. A Mumbai-style attack with marauding terrorists using high-powered weapons running through a city and creating multiple mass-casualty sites is an extreme example of the dynamics of a tactical event.

Best Possible Outcome for the Injured and the Mission Is Desired: Save as Many People as Possible

As caregivers, you are aware of the time-essential interventions needed to maintain a life. Working within a tactical situation requires situational awareness, active and continuous triage of patients, and a multiorganizational effort to save as many casualties as possible without death or serious injury to the first responders.

Good Medicine Can Sometimes Be Bad Tactics and Bad Tactics Can Get Everyone Killed and/or Cause Mission Failure

In these scenarios, maintain the safety of the responders. For example, there is little medicine performed in the direct threat care/hot zone outside of tourniquet application, due to the risk of further injury to both the casualty and the responder. The goal is to quickly move the casualty and the caregiver(s) out of the direct threat care/hot zone into the indirect threat care/warm zone.

A Medically Correct Intervention Performed at the Wrong Time May Lead to Additional Casualties

Operating in a tactical situation requires a recalibration of medical care priorities and timing. The most complex care should be provided in the evacuation care/cold zone, as the indirect threat/warm zone could unexpectedly collapse into a direct threat/hot zone. Providing complex care in the warm zone could be dire for both the patient and the caregivers.

Response and Arrival-Scene Assessment

When responding to any type of emergency event, always consider the possibility of ASHE hazards until they can be ruled out. Be vigilant when approaching the incident to identify when things "do not look right" or are unusual. Be prepared to retreat and seek cover.

If your crew has the first eyes on the situation, provide a clear and concise report to dispatch on what you observe on arrival. Multiple patients, patients with grievous trauma, the aftermath of an explosion, or evidence of an active shooter are indications of a tactical situation. Call for additional resources, try to identify the nature of the threat, and seek to identify the direct threat/hot zone.

The direct threat/hot zone represents the highest danger to caregiver and patient. There is an immediate threat for additional injury or death. If you discover you are in the direct threat/hot zone during the initial scene assessment, leave immediately. Your first priority is to gain cover. A dead caregiver provides no lifesaving care to casualties.

> **CHECK YOUR KNOWLEDGE**
>
> **When operating in a tactical situation _____ can sometimes be _____ and cause mission failure.**
>
> a. response teams; attacked
> b. too many paramedics; uncoordinated
> c. good medicine; bad tactics
> d. EMT-level caregivers; overwhelmed

Other Elements Operating Within a Tactical Environment

There are other task-focused elements operating in a civilian tactical environment that you may encounter. Local, regional, and state response to an ASHE situation continues to evolve based on experience and best practices research.

Rescue Task Force

A rescue task force (RTF) is a unit comprised of mixed resources (often EMS and law enforcement personnel)

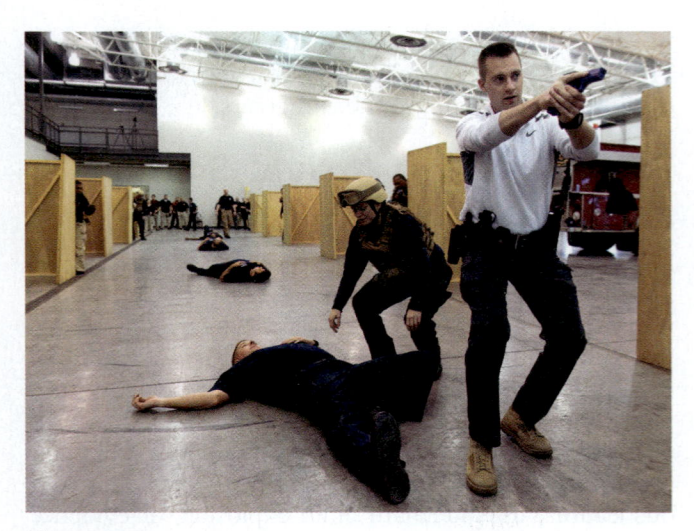

Figure 1-3 Conducting rescue task force training.
© Megan Farmer/The World-Herald/AP Images.

Tactical Emergency Medical Support

TEMS teams encompass the provision of preventive, urgent, and emergent medical care during high-risk, extended-duration, and mission-driven law enforcement special operations. EMS caregivers are embedded within the law enforcement special operations teams.

The TEMS provider serves as the tactical commander's medical conscience. The medical support unit provides the tactical commander with real-time advice and action based on situational considerations. The TEMS provider can provide a medical threat assessment of a planned operation.

At times, wounded individuals may be located in an area inaccessible to direct medical care. Remote medical assessment and TEMS-directed self-care are responsibilities of the tactical EMS caregiver.

who work together to provide point-of-wound care to tactical casualties while tactical EMS works to provide assessment and treatment to responders.

The RTF approach starts with the assumption that the entire building is a direct threat/hot zone. The goal of law enforcement is to immediately locate the shooter or shooters and neutralize the threat as soon as possible, using all of the available resources. During this effort, law enforcement is securing sections of the building. Once a section is secured by law enforcement, it becomes an indirect threat/warm zone. EMS caregivers join law enforcement in the indirect threat/warm zones to locate and treat casualties.

The goal for EMS caregivers is to treat life-threatening conditions, stabilize casualties, and rapidly remove casualties from the indirect threat/warm zone into the cold zone. Injured casualties are treated as they are reached by EMS caregivers; there is no triage. People who can walk without assistance are directed to self-evacuate down a cleared corridor under law enforcement direction (within the warm zones) (**Figure 1-3**).

> **CHECK YOUR KNOWLEDGE**
>
> _____ focuses on medical care of the first responders.
>
> a. Medical branch
> b. Tactical emergency medical support
> c. Rescue task force
> d. Police medic

Summary

The NAEMT TECC course will provide you with a set of best-practice treatment guidelines for trauma care in the high-threat prehospital environment. The course content is developed to provide care for all patients in a civilian tactical environment.

REFERENCES AND RESOURCES

National Association of Emergency Medical Technicians. *PHTLS: Prehospital Trauma Life Support*. 9th ed. Burlington, MA: Public Safety Group; 2019.

The National Academies of Sciences, Engineering, Medicine. Up to 20 percent of U.S. trauma deaths could be prevented with better care; integration of military and civilian trauma care systems needed to reach national aim of zero preventable deaths after injury. June 17, 2016. http://www8.nationalacademies.org/onpinews/newsitem.aspx?RecordID=23511. Accessed December 6, 2018.

LESSON 2

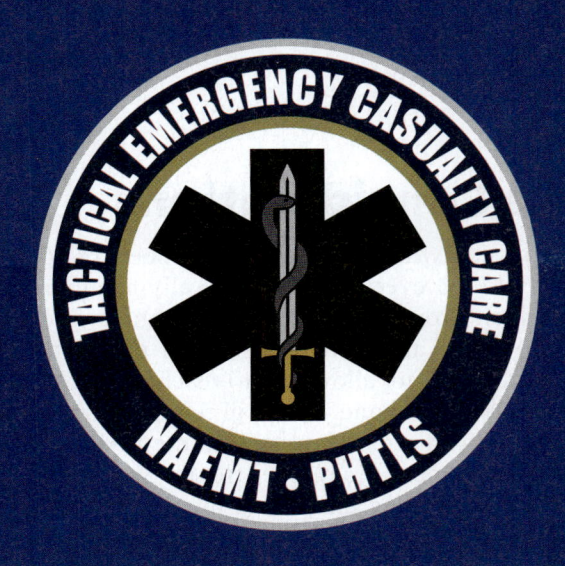

Direct Threat Care/Hot Zone

LESSON OBJECTIVES
- Define characteristics of a direct threat environment/hot zone.
- Discuss the rationale for limited medical interventions during a direct threat.
- Discuss how mission tempo and skill sets impact provider action during the direct threat phase.
- Identify drag and carry techniques.
- Discuss military experience with tourniquets and review the mechanism of action, placement, and optimization techniques for tourniquet use in direct threat care.

Direct Threat Care/Hot Zone

Lesson 2: Direct Threat Care/Hot Zone focuses on tactical emergency casualty care (TECC) operations within the direct threat/hot zone. This zone represents the highest danger to caregiver and patient as there is an immediate threat of additional injury or death and the incident scene is not secure. The emphasis in this zone is on threat suppression, preventing further casualties, extracting casualties from the high-threat area, and implementing control of life-threatening extremity hemorrhage.

Operating in the Direct Threat Care/Hot Zone

Events that require a TECC response are unpredictable and evolve quickly. Caregivers should anticipate that they are responding to a dynamic situation until an on-scene situational assessment is completed. Examples of direct threat/hot zone conditions include an active shooter with a clear field of fire, working within a crumbling building, operating within a blast range of an explosive device, or being too close to a radiation source or hazardous material. In addition, sometimes a safe incident scene may become unsafe.

Very little medical care is provided in the direct threat/hot zone. The emphasis is on identifying the threats, making direct threat/hot zone areas into indirect threat/warm zones, and removing savable casualties to evacuation/cold zone areas.

Get Off the X

An immediate objective for caregivers working in a direct threat/hot zone is to "get off the X." The X is the area where a provider is currently standing, sitting, walking, or working that might be a target for the threat (e.g., in a sniper's line of fire or within the blast zone of an undetonated device). For TECC, getting off the X means mitigating the cause of the direct threat or moving the patient and caregivers to a safer area. EMS crews working around the civil disturbances in Ferguson, Missouri, were challenged with an X that kept moving. That is, they would be operating in the cold zone tending to a patient in a home; when carrying that patient to the ambulance, they would suddenly find themselves in a direct threat/hot zone because the rioters had moved.

Constantly Changing Threat Environment

The after-action analysis of tactical situations shows that until all threats are identified and neutralized, the incident scene will remain dynamic, with sudden changes in the location of threats and identification of direct threat/hot zones and indirect threat/warm zones. This will require an immediate response from TECC caregivers in moving out of direct threat/hot zones.

Controlling life-threatening extremity hemorrhage is the only clinical care objective in the direct threat/hot zone. Because the other objective is to extract casualties from the high-threat area, the care given needs to be quick and allow for rapid patient movement.

Providing additional care in the indirect threat/warm zone may be interrupted if the area suddenly becomes a direct threat care/hot zone. Patients and TECC caregivers need to immediately move out of the direct threat care zone.

Cover Versus Concealment

Getting off the X may mean seeking cover or concealment. *Cover* is anything that will stop bullets. A concrete wall, a telephone pole, a car's engine block—these are all places where you can hide and know that a bullet will not pass through to you. It can be said that cover hides and protects you from a bullet.

Concealment does not stop bullets. These are things like hollow-core wooden doors, wooden fences, and vehicle doors. A bullet will pass through all of these and has the potential to hit you. All concealment does is hide you from sight. Keep in mind that all cover is concealment, because it hides you from both bullets and from sight, but not all concealment is cover (**Figure 2-1**).

Mitigation of Direct Threats

The goal of a tactical casualty situation is to accomplish the mission (mitigating the threat) with minimal casualties and to prevent any casualty from sustaining additional injuries. Threat mitigation techniques are used to neutralize the existing threat, such as an active shooter, confined space, hazardous materials, or unstable structure. The objective is rapid casualty access and egress.

In-depth medical intervention is delayed until the patient is out of the direct threat/hot zone. The medical focus is on stopping life-threatening external hemorrhage. The tactical focus is to move the casualty from the direct threat/hot zone into the indirect threat/warm zone. Any patient who is a law enforcement officer or other first responder is directed to stay engaged in any tactical operation that may occur in this zone. If able, the patient is directed to move to a safer position and apply self-aid.

> ### CHECK YOUR KNOWLEDGE
> **The zone that represents the highest danger to caregiver and patient is the _____ zone.**
> a. tactical
> b. direct threat
> c. indirect threat
> d. evacuation care

Rescue Considerations

Each TECC mission will have a tempo, or speed, of activities. Many TECC events start chaotically as emergency responders from multiple organizations arrive, assess the situation, and initiate an action plan. The tactical situation may not allow you to reach a casualty in the direct threat/hot zone. This will require what is known as a rapid and remote assessment methodology (RAM) and development of a rescue attempt plan. RAM is the process of assessing and rendering aid to those who are out of direct physical and visual contact of the provider. Providing emergency medical care to patients in a direct threat/hot zone environment is challenging for numerous reasons, including the lack of advanced diagnostic tools, limited supplies, the probability of severe injuries, austere environments, and the unique complexities of being under fire. Caregivers must be flexible, with the ability to adapt to unexpected situations and perform a remote medical assessment, which involves assessing a patient without being able to visualize the patient. Binoculars, robots, and video cameras are some of the technologies available.

Rapid and Remote Assessment Methodology

Remote medical assessments are based on the RAM developed by the Counter Narcotics and Terrorism Operational Medical Support (CONTOMS) program at the Uniformed Services University of the Health Sciences, the U.S. Department of Defense's medical school. The principal purpose of this assessment algorithm is to maximize the opportunity to extract and treat a salvageable casualty while minimizing risk to TEMS providers from attempting an unnecessary rescue, and the algorithm is most applicable during the direct threat/hot zone phase of care (**Figure 2-2**). Unnecessary rescues fall into two categories: (1) those in which the casualty can extract himself or herself, and (2) those in which the casualty is already dead (more appropriately termed a "body recovery"). The RAM provides an organized approach to evaluate the totality of circumstances from a protected position before recommending a rescue attempt to the commander or authority having jurisdiction.

The first step in conducting a remote assessment is to determine if the area is secure. If it is, standard EMS care is appropriate after ensuring that the casualty cannot harm tactical emergency medical support (TEMS) providers. If the area is not secure, use available intelligence to determine whether the casualty is a perpetrator or otherwise represents a threat. Under such circumstances, *no further medical intervention is indicated until the threat has been controlled*. To do otherwise

LESSON 2 Direct Threat Care/Hot Zone

might jeopardize the safety of tactical officers, emergency medical services (EMS) providers, and innocent parties. If the casualty is not deemed a perpetrator, a remote assessment should be initiated to attempt to evaluate the nature of the injury and the stability of the casualty's condition.

Remote observation is the first technique to be employed during the remote assessment because it allows EMS providers to gather information without revealing their position or intent to the hostile force. Technology available to special weapons and tactics (SWAT) teams can improve the reliability of this assessment. For example, a good pair of binoculars or night-vision goggles can often help to ascertain if the casualty is breathing, the rate and quality of respirations, the presence of life-threatening hemorrhage, and the presence of obvious wounds incompatible with life. In cold weather, a respiratory condensation plume can often be seen from the casualty's mouth if the casualty is breathing. Acoustic surveillance equipment, if available, can be deployed to detect speech, moans, groans, and even respiratory sounds. Thermal imaging technology has improved in recent years and may be considered for application in the RAM. If such technology is not available, a simple remote visual assessment should be performed.

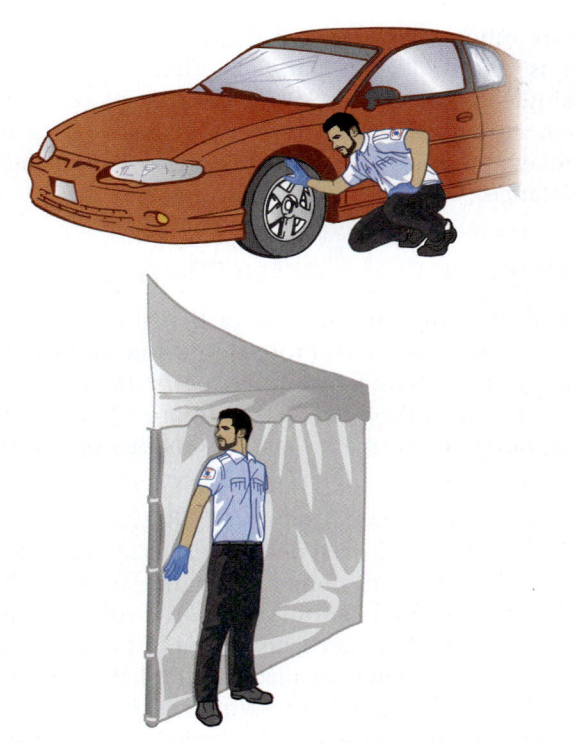

Figure 2-1 The difference between concealment and cover.
Courtesy CPL Matt Cain Ventura Police Department.

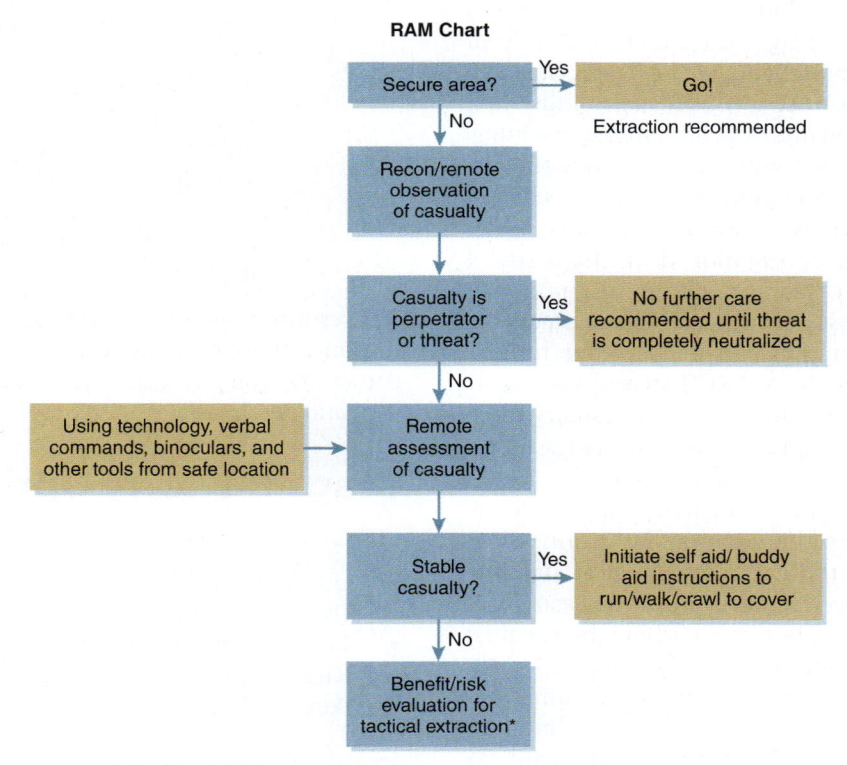

*The benefit/risk evaluation of tactical extraction will depend on the likelihood of survival of casualty. The decision will ultimately be made by the SWAT commander with significant medical input from the TEMS provider.

Figure 2-2 Rapid and remote assessment methodology (RAM) flowchart.
© National Association of Emergency Medical Technicians (NAEMT).

If communication is possible with the patient or someone next to the patient, the caregiver must be able to ask questions and give instructions using simple and concise language, taking special care to avoid complexity. Three competencies are critical. These include (1) the ability to remain calm, (2) to avoid the use of medical jargon, and (3) to complete a head-to-toe assessment using another's eyes, ears, and hands. Caregivers must first introduce themselves, their partner, and provide calm reassurance. The caregiver asks the casualty or person next to the casualty his or her name or how he or she is to be addressed, and if he or she has any prior medical or first aid training. Next, the caregiver should ask for a quick overview of the state and position of the patient, keeping in mind the MARCH assessment protocol. The MARCH sequence is a key assessment in TECC and is covered in further detail later. In performing a remote assessment, MARCH uses the following sequence of assessment areas:

- M Massive hemorrhage control
- A Airway patency
- R Respiratory status
- C Circulatory status
- H Hypothermia/Head injury

Key considerations include whether the patient is injured or ill, presence of significant bleeding, state of breathing, presence of pulse, and level of consciousness. The casualty or person next to the casualty must first treat any life-threatening injuries with emergency interventions, such as applying tourniquets, opening the airway, and/or occluding open chest wounds, as needed.

The ability to improvise materials may save a life. The caregiver must get information from the casualty or person next to the casualty regarding the presence of medical supplies, first aid kits, and other accessible nonmedical equipment that can be used for tourniquets and splints. After the MARCH survey and treatment, the casualty or person next to the casualty must be coached through a rapid head-to-toe assessment, noting as many physical findings as possible.

A tactical extraction of the casualty may be determined to be optimal by the commander at any time, but the situation, not the casualty's medical stability, should primarily inform this decision. If the casualty is unstable, the risk of extraction must be weighed against the benefits of immediate access to medical care. Although this is a command decision, the commander will rely heavily on the TEMS provider's assessment of the patient's condition and the need for immediate extraction. If the benefit–risk ratio is sufficiently high, the extraction may proceed.

Although the algorithm seems logical, it is crucial to have a decision structure that fosters good assessment before emotion overtakes reason and a needless rescue is risked. The military experience is filled with examples of numerous casualties that were incurred in an attempt to recover a body or rescue a casualty who eventually stood up and ran to cover without assistance.

Operational Performance

A comprehensive approach to tactical situations can be found in National Fire Protection Association (NFPA) 3000 (PS): *Standard for an Active Shooter/Hostile Event Response (ASHER) Program,* 2018 Edition. NFPA describes operational performance as a combination of three factors:

1. Resource availability/reliability. Are the trained and specialized personnel easily available and ready to respond? Depending on one official to go to a central warehouse to open up the mass-trauma cache may not be considered an immediately available and reliable resource.
2. Agency capability. What is the organization's ability to effectively deploy and manage an active shooter or hostile event incident? Each successive event creates lessons learned for that agency as well as others.
3. Operational effectiveness. This is determined by the skills and readiness of the teams. For example, the 1995 bombing of the Murrah Building in Oklahoma City was the first time all of the federally funded urban search and rescue teams were deployed together. Some teams had years of local and international experience, and others were on their first mission.

The resources (personnel and equipment) needed for the response must be considered versus the potential outcomes, including civilian injury and death, responder injury and death, and property loss.

Drag and Carry Options

TECC covers five drag and carry options:

- One-person drag
- Two-person drag
- Two-person side-by-side carry
- Pack strap/Hawes carry
- Fore/aft carry

One-Person Drag

The one-person drag is the most appropriate to move a person with multiple injuries who cannot walk or is unconscious. The caregiver drags the patient by pulling on the clothing in the neck and shoulder area. To perform this drag, grab clothing just behind the collar, use your arms to support the patient's head, and drag the patient out of the direct threat/hot zone (**Figure 2-3**).

Two-Person Drag

The two-person drag is similar to the one-person drag (**Figure 2-4**). In this case, two caregivers each grasp the clothing with one hand to rapidly remove the casualty to safety. The caregivers should make every reasonable effort to keep the spine in alignment with the neck and head.

Two-Person Side-by-Side Carry

Caregivers cradle the patient between them in the two-person side-by-side carry (**Figure 2-5**).

- Start by kneeling beside the patient near the patient's hips.
- Raise the patient to a sitting position; the caregivers link arms behind the patient's back.
- Caregivers place their free arms under the patient's knees and link arms.
- If possible, the patient places his or her arms around the necks of the caregivers.

Pack Strap/Hawes Carry

Do not use the pack strap/Hawes carry if the patient has a fractured wrist or arm (**Figure 2-6**). Using it with an unconscious patient requires a second caregiver to help position the injured or ill person on your back.

- Have the patient stand or have a second responder support the person.
- Position yourself with your back to the person, back straight, knees bent, so that your shoulders fit into the person's armpits.

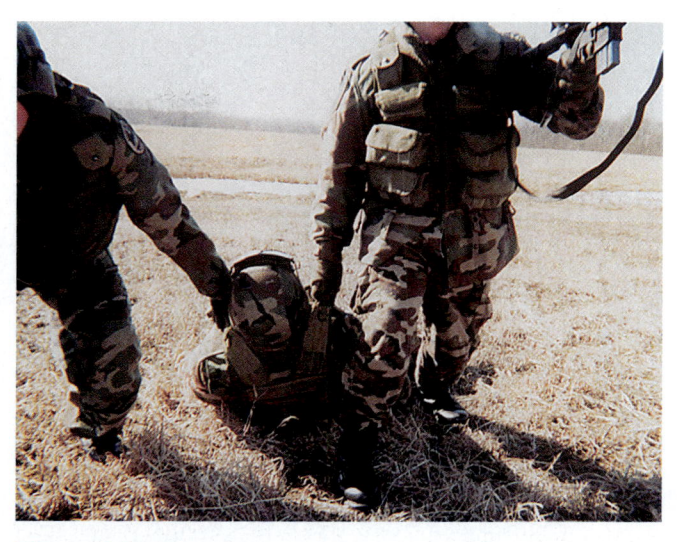

Figure 2-4 Two-person drag.
Courtesy of Dr. Mel Otten.

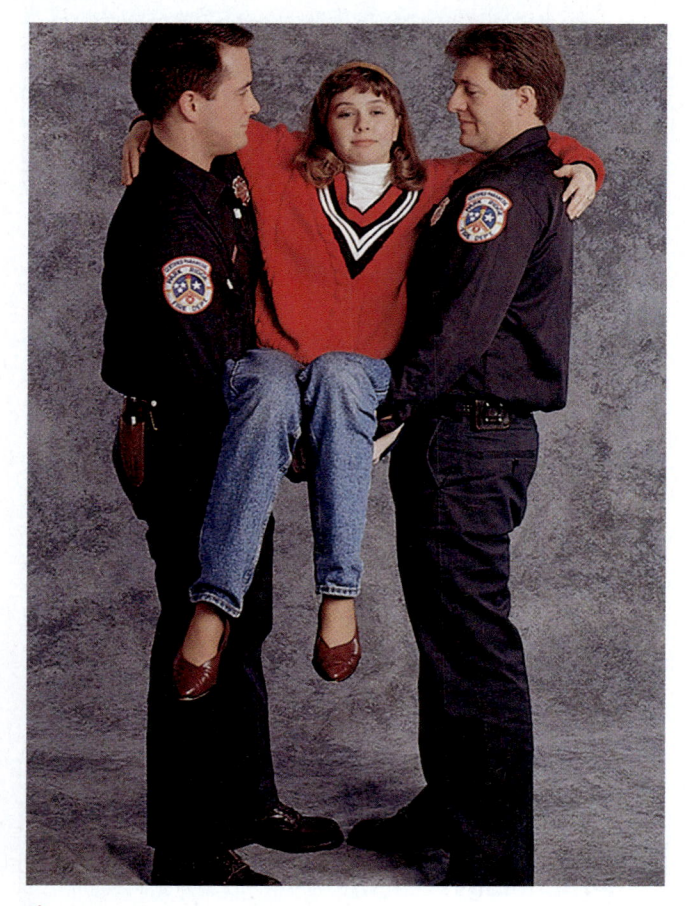

Figure 2-5 Side-by-side carry.
© Jones & Bartlett Learning. Courtesy of MIEMSS.

- Cross the person's arms in front of you and grasp the person's wrists. Lean forward slightly and pull the person up and onto your back. Stand up and walk to safety.

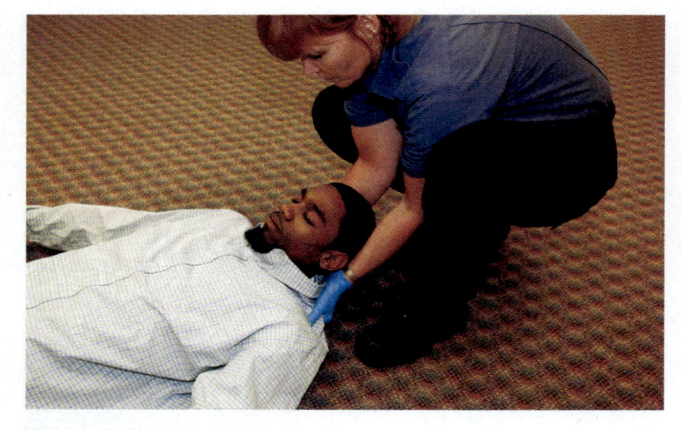

Figure 2-3 One-person drag.
© Jones & Bartlett Learning. Courtesy of MIEMSS.

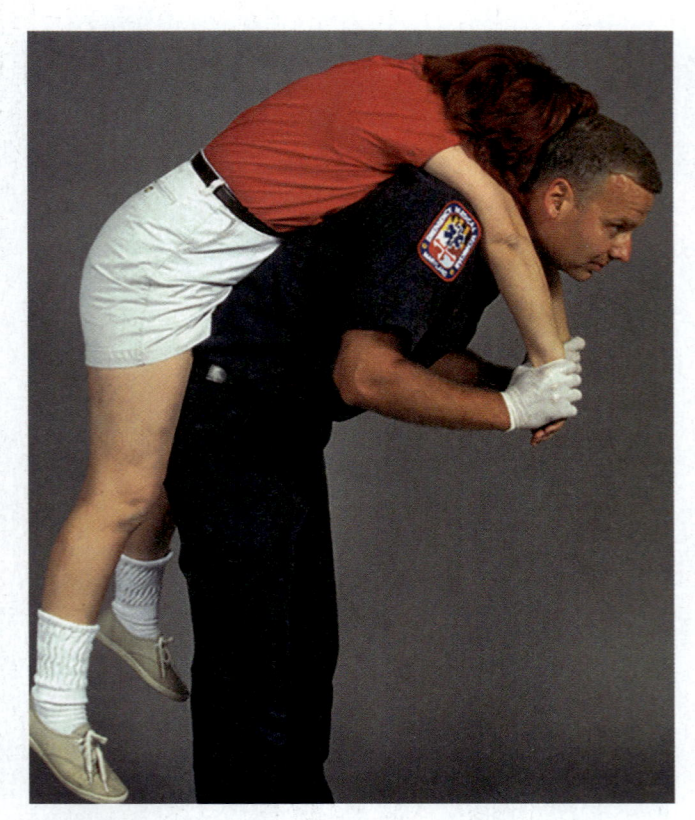

Figure 2-6 Pack strap/Hawes carry.
© Jones & Bartlett Learning. Courtesy of MIEMSS.

- Depending on the size of the person, you may be able to hold both of his or her wrists with one hand, leaving your other hand free to help maintain balance, open doors, and remove obstructions.

Fore/Aft Carry

Two caregivers are required for the fore/aft carry. One caregiver grasps the patient's legs and one caregiver grasps the patient's forearms/wrists by reaching under the armpits from behind. The caregivers simultaneously raise the patient and begin the carry.

> **CHECK YOUR KNOWLEDGE**
>
> **Which is a key factor of remote assessment methodology?**
> a. The caregiver is embedded with the casualty until the direct threat is mitigated.
> b. The caregiver is unable to get direction from online medical control.
> c. The caregiver is unable to touch the patient.
> d. Sending live video from the direct threat/hot zone to the medical sector

Medical Interventions in the Direct Threat Care/ Hot Zone

Place Patient in the Recovery Position

A TECC caregiver in the direct threat/hot zone may only have the time to place the patient in the recovery position. This is a variant of the three-quarters prone position of the body. This position will passively maintain an open airway and allow vomit, blood, and secretions to drain from the upper airway (**Figure 2-7**).

Controlling Massive Hemorrhage

The only other medical intervention that takes place within the direct threat/hot zone is to control massive hemorrhage. Exsanguination, the process of draining or losing critical blood volume, and hemorrhage, an escape of blood from a ruptured blood vessel, especially when profuse, account for the greatest proportion of trauma deaths in the prehospital setting. Hemorrhage is also responsible for the largest number of trauma-related fatalities within the first hour of arrival at a trauma center, 80% of operating room deaths, and 50% of deaths within the first 24 hours of definitive trauma care.

Arterial hemorrhage, particularly when it occurs proximal to the distal third of an extremity, or any complicated arterial or severe venous hemorrhage associated with a mangled limb, represents an immediate life threat. Apply direct pressure to the wound or direct the casualty or person next to them to apply pressure. Then have the patient or the person next to them apply an effective tourniquet.

If the bleeding is life threatening, a tourniquet should be placed "high and tight" in the groin or armpit above the injury, directly on the skin and free of any clothing. It should be placed as snugly as possible, with as much slack removed from the tail as possible before

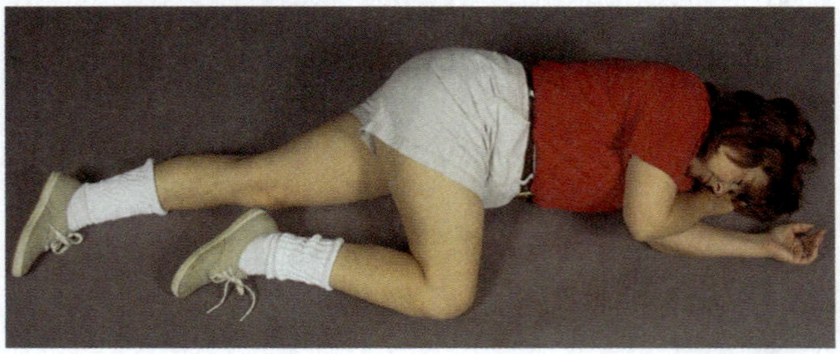

Figure 2-7 Recovery position.
© Jones & Bartlett Learning. Courtesy of MIEMSS.

the windlass is tightened. No more than three revolutions (540 degrees) of the windlass should be performed to avoid deforming the chassis of the device. In the event that one tourniquet does not stop the bleeding, it is acceptable and highly recommended to use additional tourniquets side by side until bleeding is controlled, as this provides compression of the artery over a wider area.

Types of Tourniquets

Combat Application Tourniquet

The Combat Application Tourniquet (CAT) is an effective tool to help control severe blood loss from the body's extremities. The CAT comprises five components (**Figure 2-8**):

- Friction adapter buckle
- Windlass rod
- Windlass clip
- Windlass strap
- Omni-tape (self-adhering) band

Special Operations Forces Tactical Tourniquet (SOFTT)

Both the SOFTT Gen 4 and the SOFTT Wide are strap-and-windlass tourniquets that mimic the function of a traditional tourniquet (**Figure 2-9**).

1. Pull the tourniquet over the limb and position it between the wound and the body, 2 to 4 inches from the edge of the wound site.
2. Position the strap's end to face the midline of your or the casualty's midline and tighten the strap.
3. Twist the aluminum windlass until the hemorrhage is controlled.
4. Place one end of the windlass into the triangular clip that is on the tourniquet.
5. Tighten the safety screw.

Emergency and Military Tourniquet (Pneumatic)

This pneumatic tourniquet functions like a blood pressure cuff. One difference is the reinforced air bladder and clamp that is used to secure the inflated tourniquet. The design of the device is to maintain pressure on the limb once the clamp is locked down, closing the connection between the bladder and the hand pump. It scores well in tourniquet effectiveness studies but is more expensive, bulkier, and heavier than the windlass-style devices (**Figure 2-10**).

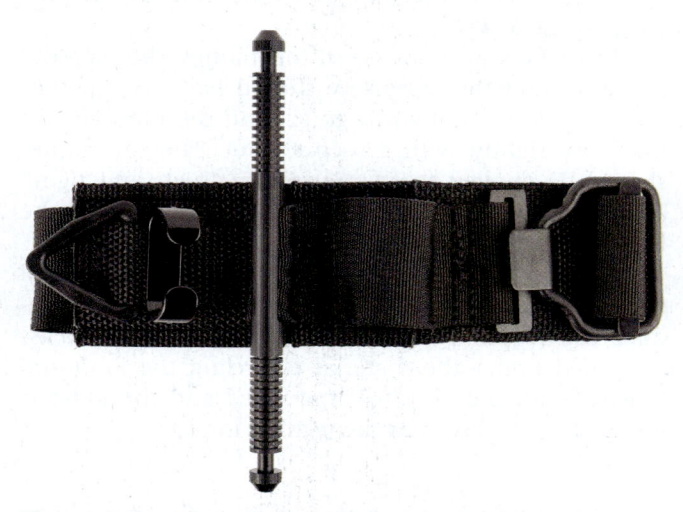

Figure 2-9 Special Operations Forces Tactical Tourniquet (SOFTT) 4th generation.
Courtesy of TacMed Solutions.

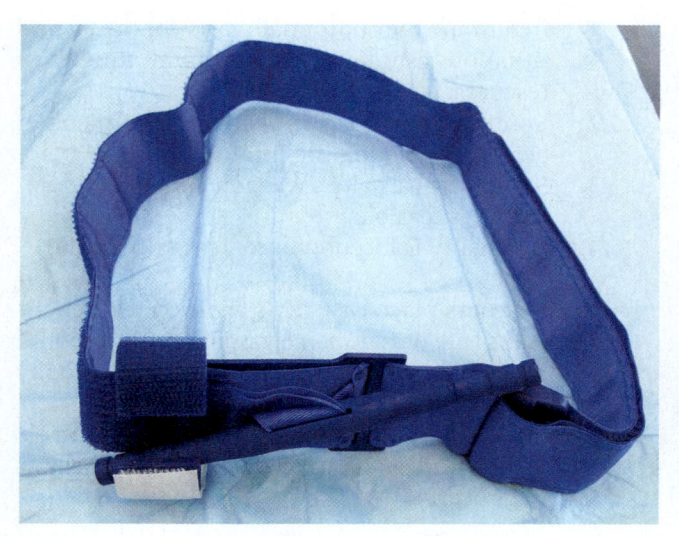

Figure 2-8 Combat Application Tourniquet (CAT).
Courtesy of Peter T. Pons, MD, FACEP.

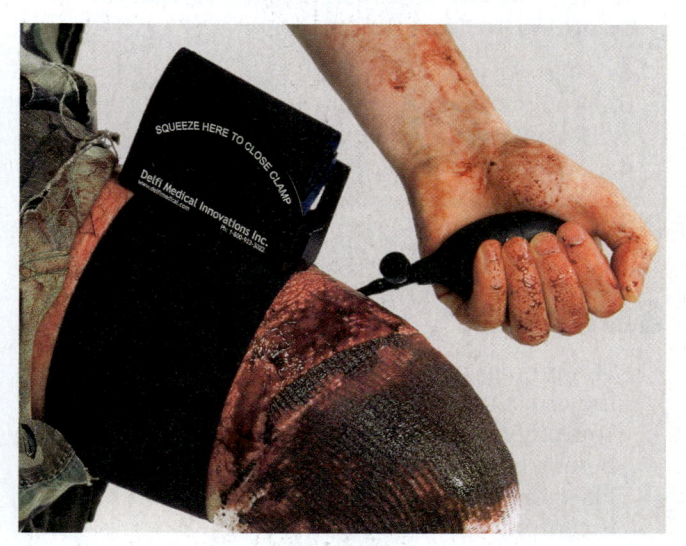

Figure 2-10 Emergency and military tourniquet.
Reproduced with permission from Emergency & Military Tourniquet, Delfi Medical. Retrieved from http://www.delfimedical.com/emergency-military-tourniquet/

```
Use only                Put it on       The tourniquet         Use a second
for potential    →     "high and        should eliminate  →    tourniquet if
life-threatening        tight."         the distal pulse and   needed.
hemorrhage.                             stop the bleeding.
```

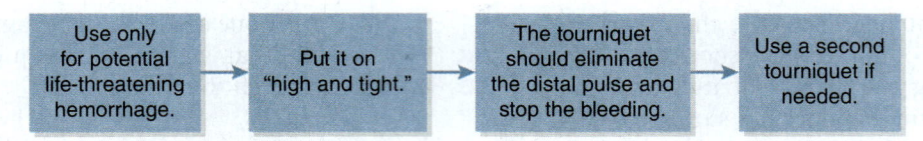

Figure 2-11 Tourniquet pearls.

Improvised Tourniquet

Tourniquets work by creating circumferential pressure around a limb that is greater than the systolic pressure present in the vessels running perpendicular to the tourniquet. Applying a tourniquet proximal to the site of bleeding serves to prevent further blood flow into the exposed limb, thereby preventing ongoing hemorrhage (**Figure 2-11**).

In making an improvised tourniquet, the material going around the extremity should be 2 to 3 inches wide and long enough to go around the limb and be tied very tightly with a secure knot. The tourniquet should be applied to the extremity "high and tight" above the wound site at the level of the groin in the lower extremity and the axilla in the upper extremity.

A windlass is used to tighten the material. You will need a rigid object of 6 to 8 inches in length to produce the required mechanical leverage. The windlass is slipped under the material encircling the limb and twisted until the bleeding is stopped and the pulse is gone. The windlass must be secured in place.

> **CHECK YOUR KNOWLEDGE**
>
> **What is the quickest medical intervention while operating in direct threat/hot zone?**
>
> a. Hemorrhage control
> b. Rapid extrication
> c. Passive airway maintenance
> d. Tactical hypotension

Summary

- The primary tactical goal is to get casualties out of the direct threat/hot zone (move off the X).
- Tourniquets are immediately used for uncontrolled hemorrhage.
- Place casualties in recovery position after bleeding is controlled.

Skill Stations

Casualty Drags and Carries

One-Person Drag

1. Determine the appropriate carry for the tactical situation, estimated distance, and number of rescuers. This drag is for short distances. This drag can be high or low profile.
2. Secure the casualty's weapon, as feasible.
3. Grasp the casualty by equipment with one or two hands.
4. Begin the drag.

Two-Person Drag

1. Determine the appropriate carry for the tactical situation, estimated distance, and number of rescuers. This drag can be high or low profile.
2. Communicate the plan with the team member before attempting the drag.
3. Secure the casualty's weapon and other equipment, as feasible.
4. Each member secures the casualty by equipment with one hand.
5. Begin the drag.

Two-Person Side-by-Side Carry

1. Determine the appropriate carry for the tactical situation, estimated distance, and number of rescuers.
2. Communicate the plan with the team member before attempting the lift.
3. Secure the casualty's weapon and other equipment, as feasible.
4. If casualty is facedown, roll casualty to the back.
5. Rescuers place casualty's arms over rescuers' necks with outside hand grasping casualty's wrist.
6. Rescuers use inside hands to secure casualty by belt, pants, or body armor.
7. Simultaneously raise casualty.
8. Step forward with casualty's feet dragging behind.
9. Begin carry.

Pack Strap/Hawes Carry

1. Determine the appropriate carry for the tactical situation, estimated distance, and number of rescuers.
2. Secure the casualty's weapon, as feasible.
3. If the casualty is able, have the casualty wrap his/her arms around the rescuer's neck.
4. The rescuer reaches over casualty's arm and grasps casualty's opposite arm just above the elbow.
5. Begin the carry.

Fore/Aft Carry

1. Determine the appropriate carry for the tactical situation, estimated distance, and number of rescuers.
2. Communicate the plan with the team member before attempting the lift.
3. Secure the casualty's weapon and other equipment, as feasible.
4. If the casualty is facedown, roll casualty to the back, and raise casualty to a sitting position.
5. One rescuer grasps casualty's legs and one rescuer grasps casualty's forearms/wrists by reaching under armpits from behind.
6. Simultaneously raise casualty.
7. Begin carry.

Tourniquet Application

1. Remove the CAT or SOFTT from the carrying pouch.
2. Slide the extremity through the loop of the self-adhering band, or wrap the self-adhering band around the extremity and reattach to the friction adapter buckle.
3. Position the tourniquet at the level of the groin in the lower extremity or the level of the axilla in the upper extremity.
4. Secure the tourniquet.
   - If applying to a leg wound, the self-adhering band must be routed through both sides of the friction adapter buckle and fastened back on itself. This will prevent it from loosening when twisting the windlass clip or tri-ring (CAT Generation 6 or older only).
5. Twist the windlass rod until the bleeding stops. When the tactical situation permits, ensure that the distal pulse is no longer palpable.
6. Lock the rod in place with the windlass clip or tri-ring.
   NOTE: For added security (and always before moving the casualty), secure the windlass rod with the windlass strap. For smaller extremities, continue to wind the self-adhering band across the windlass clip and secure it under the windlass strap.
7. Grasp the windlass strap, pull it tight, and adhere it to the Velcro on the windlass clip (CAT only).
8. The date and time of the tourniquet's application is recorded when tactically feasible.
   NOTE: The tactical situation and local protocols dictate how a wound to a real casualty is dressed and whether the casualty would be transported to definitive treatment.

REFERENCES AND RESOURCES

Callaway DW. Emergency medical services in disasters. Hogan DE, Burstein JL, eds. *Disaster Medicine*. 2nd ed. Philadelphia, PA: Lippincott, Williams and Wilkins; 2016:127-139.

Cloonan C. *Proceedings of the Third International Conference on Tactical Emergency Medical Support*. Bethesda, MD: Uniformed Services University of the Health Sciences; 1999.

Fisher AD, Will G. Next generation combat medic. Buyer beware: selecting your next everyday carry tourniquet. https://nextgencombatmedic.com/2017/09/14/buyer-beware-selecting-your-everyday-carry-tourniquet/. September 14, 2017. Accessed December 6, 2018.

Kragh JF, O'Neill ML, Walters TJ, Dubick MA, Baer DG, Wade CE, Holcomb JB, Blackbourne LH. The military emergency tourniquet program's lessons learned with devices and designs. *Mil Med*. 2011;176(10):1144-1152.

Mack M, Springer B, Ten Eyck R. Medicine across the barricade. *MedEdPORTAL*. 2013;9:9332.

McKay S, Hoyne S. High threat immediate extraction: the Immediate Reaction Team (IRT) model. *Tactical Edge*. Spring 2007:50-54.

National Association of Emergency Medical Technicians. *PHTLS: Prehospital Trauma Life Support*. 9th ed. Burlington, MA: Public Safety Group; 2019.

National Fire Protection Association. *NFPA 300 (PS): Standard for an Active Shooter/Hostile Event Response (ASHER) Program*. Quincy, MA: NFPA; 2018.

Shackelford SA, Butler FK Jr, Kragh JF Jr, et al. Optimizing the use of limb tourniquets in tactical combat casualty care: TCCC guidelines change 14-02. *J Spec Op Med*. 2015;15(1):17-31.

LESSON 3

Indirect Threat Care/Warm Zone: MARCH—Patient Assessment and Massive Hemorrhage Interventions

LESSON OBJECTIVES
- Discuss the dynamic transition from direct threat care to indirect threat care.
- Describe the need for weapon removal from casualties with altered mental status.
- Identify steps in the MARCH assessment.
- Explain the Primary, Alternative, Contingency, Emergency (PACE) methodology.
- Demonstrate the most appropriate hemorrhage control method based on physical assessment and resources.
- Demonstrate safe and effective application of junctional tourniquets and in anatomic locations not amenable to tourniquet placement.
- Demonstrate safe and effective application of pressure dressings and hemostatic dressings.

Indirect Threat Care/Warm Zone

Indirect threat care/warm zone involves providing definitive lifesaving medical interventions in an area of relative safety that has been cleared but not secured. That means that there still is an unmitigated threat, it is just not imminent.

The dynamic nature of a tactical situation means that the indirect threat care/warm zone is not a fixed area. This zone could quickly deteriorate into a direct threat/hot zone due to movement of an active shooter, identification of another life threat, structural instability, rapid fire development, or explosion. While operating in the indirect threat/warm zone, the tactical emergency casualty care (TECC) provider should be alert to changes in the safety of the situation and be prepared to immediately move to a more secure area.

Your first patient encounter may be in the indirect threat/warm zone or with a patient who was quickly removed from the direct threat/hot zone. Patients evacuated from the direct threat care/hot zone may have either received no medical interventions or received only an initial intervention to control massive hemorrhage.

Scene Safety

Providing patient care in the warm zone requires a constant risk–benefit analysis, as well as situational awareness of the surroundings and the clinical condition of the patient. A vital component of operating in the indirect threat/warm zone is ensuring and relying on joint command and control by all disciplines involved at an incident.

Active shooter events that are unmitigated provide a particularly dangerous situation, as the shooter or shooters could remain mobile. Caregivers may find themselves suddenly operating "on the X," that is, within a direct threat/hot zone, when the active shooter moves. That means caregivers need to work as part of a larger team, with no freelancing. This will also help prevent friendly fire incidents.

Mass-casualty events may require technical rescue resources to force open doors and breech walls to rescue and extract casualties. For example, during the 2016 Pulse nightclub event, the Orlando special weapons and tactics (SWAT) team breached the rear wall to establish an exit path for trapped club-goers. Fire, rescue, and EMS personnel should utilize their breaching and rescue experience in a collaborative effort to rescue and extract casualties when developing egress options from the indirect threat/warm zone. Establish the safest and quickest path to get from the indirect threat/warm zone into the evacuation/cold zone.

Asymmetrical Response

You may need to consider an "asymmetrical" rescue path to increase provider safety and the speed of extraction. That is, the most direct and safest route may not be along conventional corridors or be the most obvious route. For instance, is a window more expedient than a door? You should look for hasty but effective extraction routes while keeping away from threats and maintaining cover. Recall that the way you went in may not be the best way to exit.

Actions must be communicated and coordinated with the unified command to avoid friendly fire or unintended consequences (**Figure 3-1**).

Threat Management

Two special situations require a specific response by TECC caregivers during an operation. Injured law enforcement and military officers with altered mental status should have their weapons and communications equipment secured by the appropriate authorities. Altered mental status may be due to shock, hypoxia, traumatic brain injury, and pain medications. In the chaotic "fog of response," an armed responder suffering from an altered level of consciousness is a safety and operational hazard. That is, the armed responder may interpret the caregiver's actions as a life-threatening assault and may respond with deadly force. In this situation, the appropriate and authorized agency representative should secure the casualty's weapons and communications equipment (so that a responder with an altered mental status cannot communicate with incident command) (**Figure 3-2**).

Weapons and hazardous devices may be discovered during operations. Appropriate, trained, and authorized representatives should secure the weapons and devices. The role of TECC caregivers is to identify, isolate, and report discovered weapons.

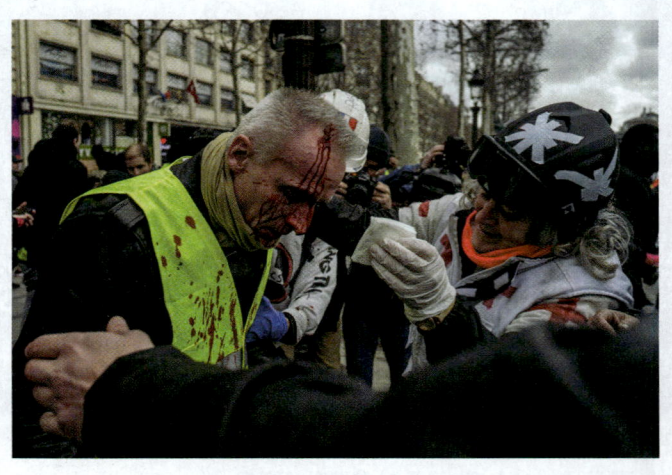

Figure 3-2 Secure weapons and communications equipment from an officer with altered mental status.
© Omar Havana/Getty Images News/Getty Images.

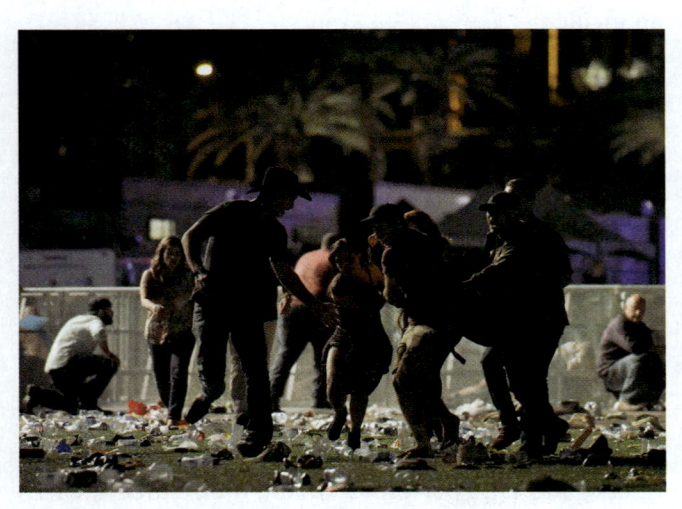

Figure 3-1 Consider "asymmetrical" rescue to increase provider safety and speed of extraction.
© David Becker/Getty Images News/Getty Images.

> **CHECK YOUR KNOWLEDGE**
>
> **Deploying a fire company hose line to obscure or interfere with an active shooter's line-of-sight is an example of:**
>
> a. freelancing.
> b. responding with overwhelming response.
> c. asymmetric response.
> d. fortifying the rescue corridor.

Assessment and Intervention Priorities

The MARCH assessment and treatment protocol is a core element of TECC. It is a simple acronym for remembering the necessary steps in priority for saving lives after a blast or penetrating injuries: **M**assive hemorrhage, **A**irway, **R**espiratory, **C**irculation, and **H**ead/Hypothermia.

The MARCH protocol provides a patient assessment and treatment map. The goal of the MARCH protocol is to delay a casualty from dying long enough to receive hospital-level care. After the 75th Ranger Regiment of the U.S. Army Special Operations Command was trained in Tactical Combat Casualty Care (TCCC) and the MARCH assessment, the number of preventable deaths on the battlefield dropped from the service-wide average of 24% to 3%. Stopping massive hemorrhage saved lives.

Bleeding Assessment

The first step in the MARCH assessment is to identify massive hemorrhage. This assessment starts as you walk up to the patient. If the patient is conscious, explain what you are about to do. Scan the area to identify weapons that may be in the patient's hands or within immediate reach. Visually identify all hemorrhage sources. The patient may be lying on the major source of hemorrhage or it may be hidden by the patient's clothes. Wounds that damage major blood vessels (subclavian, axillary, brachial, radial, carotid, femoral, or popliteal) can lead to exsanguination (**Figure 3-3**).

Blood sweeps are performed by sweeping both hands over the casualty's entire body. Work from head to toe, stopping every few inches to look at your gloves for signs of blood. By stopping every few inches and checking for signs of blood, you will be able to locate the injuries quickly and address the problems they may present that much quicker. A blood sweep is most often performed in the warm zone.

Blood sweeps only work well with clean gloves, major hemorrhage, and light. A combination of raking and sweeping is more effective. *Raking* means assessing by spreading your fingers out and curving them in, resembling a rake you would you use to remove leaves from a lawn. Your fingers will detect wounds that may be missed under bloody clothes. Expose and access each wound found.

A blood sweep-and-rake assessment is similar to the emergency medical technician/paramedic physical head-to-toe secondary assessment. The tactical situation will determine how much of an assessment you can do while in the indirect threat/warm zone. The priority of the blood sweep and rake is to identify all hemorrhage locations.

- Palpate the top and back of the head first. Inspect your gloved hands for traces of blood. Observe the ears, nose, mouth, and eyes for evidence of bleeding.
- Move your gloved hands to sweep the back of the neck while observing the location and condition of the throat.

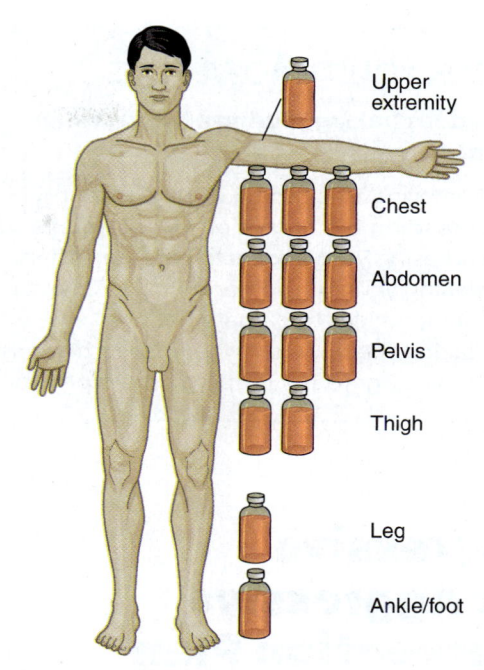

Figure 3-3 Potential blood loss from various parts of the body. Each bottle equals 1 pint (473 ml).
© Jones & Bartlett Learning.

- Just like a prehospital trauma survey, if you are in the cold zone, remove clothing if possible and palpate each arm individually. Sweep from shoulder to elbow, stopping to inspect your gloved hands for traces of blood. Continue from elbow to fingers and do a second inspection of your gloved hands.
- Inspect the central core by going back to the shoulders and palpating the chest and abdomen. If clinically appropriate and tactically possible, logroll the casualty toward you in order to visualize and palpate the back. If unable to logroll patient, palpate the back by placing your gloved hands under the patient.
- Palpate the pelvis and buttocks.
- Take each leg and individually palpate, starting from the inguinal fold and moving down to the knee, stopping to inspect your gloved hands for traces of blood. Resume palpation from the knee to the toes.

Control all hemorrhaging wounds discovered during the blood sweep-and-rake procedure. An on-scene estimate of blood loss is notably poor, with 87% of caregivers underestimating the amount of blood loss and becoming more inaccurate as the amount of blood on the ground increases. In the TECC environment the focus is on stopping the bleeding and controlling life-threatening conditions until the patient gets to hospital-level interventions.

> **CHECK YOUR KNOWLEDGE**
>
> **What does "raking" during a blood sweep mean?**
>
> a. Removing all clothing during assessment
> b. Spreading the fingers of your gloved hands and using your fingers to palpate patient
> c. Making your gloved hand into a fist and using your knuckles to palpate patient
> d. Placing the fingers of your gloved hand into a "V" and vigorously tapping on the patient

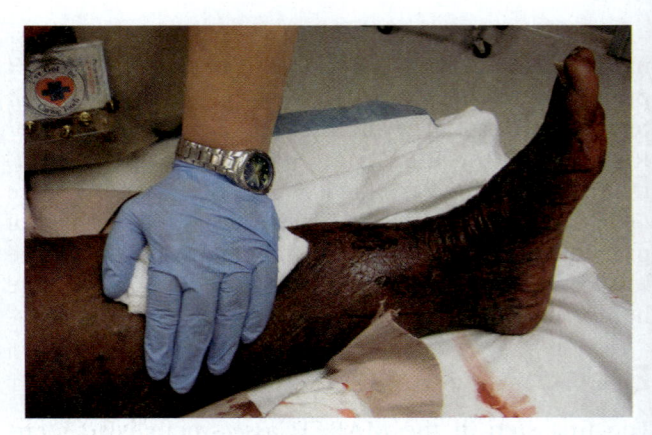

Figure 3-4 Applying direct pressure to the wound.
Courtesy of Rhonda Hunt.

Progressive and Aggressive Intervention Plan

According to the American College of Surgeons, uncontrolled bleeding is the number one cause of preventable death from trauma. Therefore, controlling hemorrhage as early as possible is a critical component of both operational medicine and trauma management. In ASHE environments, the criticality of hemorrhage control must be balanced with operational risk assessments. A planning tool that can be used when faced with clinical care needs in a tactical setting is the four-step PACE methodology. A TECC caregiver categorizes the clinical plan based on the tactical situation, patient condition, equipment available, and available staffing:

- **Primary Plan**: The preferred clinical care technique
- **Alternative Plan**: A clinical care technique that should produce the same outcome as the primary plan
- **Contingency Plan**: A backup technique that is not as effective as the primary or alternative clinical plan.
- **Emergency Plan**: When the primary, alternative, and contingency plans fail, or there is a sudden change in the tactical situation that requires an immediate evacuation. This technique is used to meet the primary objective of the clinical care goal until the TECC caregiver and the patient can get to an area of safety with more resources.

The PACE methodology can be a valuable tool for hemorrhage control.

- Primary: Tourniquet
- Alternative: Direct pressure
- Contingency: Wound packing, junctional tourniquet
- Emergency: Manual pressure until patient gets to definitive care

Tourniquets are the most effective, rapid intervention available. Hemostatic dressings require 3 to 5 minutes of continuous pressure. Other techniques and tools are described in the following sections.

Direct Pressure

The goal is to stop or significantly reduce the hemorrhagic loss of blood. Direct pressure occludes blood vessels and assists in triggering the clotting cascade (**Figure 3-4**).

Direct pressure is a temporary, yet expedient measure to stop carotid and femoral bleeding that requires more definitive care when tactically possible. Pressure must be held for at least 3 minutes before determining if it is effective. Do not release direct pressure until you are prepared to control the bleeding with additional means. Consider focusing your direct pressure on the damaged vessel or wound, using two fingers instead of the entire palm of a hand. If you do not have a free hand, or need your hands for another intervention, using your knee or elbow may work. If you must move your casualty, consider using a combination of a firm pressure dressing augmented by manual pressure.

> **CHECK YOUR KNOWLEDGE**
>
> **When using PACE methodology in hemorrhagic control, wound packing would be an example of which step?**
>
> a. Primary
> b. Alternative
> c. Contingency
> d. Emergency

Extremity Tourniquets

Rapid blood loss leads to irreversible hemorrhagic shock and exsanguination. There are four classes of hemorrhagic shock:

- Class I: Loss of up to 15% of blood volume, 750 milliliters (ml) in an adult
- Class II: Loss of 15% to 30% of blood volume, 750 ml to 1,500 ml in an adult
- Class III: Loss of 30% to 40% of blood volume, 1,500 ml to 2,000 ml in an adult
- Class IV: Loss of more than 40% of blood volume, greater than 2,000 ml in an adult

Class III patients exhibit classic signs of shock and will require fluid resuscitation once all hemorrhage sources are controlled. Class IV patients have minutes to live and require immediate control of hemorrhage and aggressive resuscitation (**Table 3-1**).

Tourniquet Optimization

A lifesaving take-away from the military's experience is that early application of tourniquets saves lives by slowing down the progression of hemorrhagic shock and exsanguination. High-velocity penetrating trauma and blast injury are common in military combat, resulting in extensive wounding and mangled extremities. TCCC Guidelines Change 14-02 cites studies by Kragh et al. that found when a tourniquet is placed early on a combat casualty, before the onset of hemorrhagic shock, there is a 10% mortality. When a tourniquet is placed after the signs of shock are present, as described in a Class III or Class IV hemorrhagic shock condition, there is a 90% mortality.

Tourniquets applied hastily over clothing in the direct threat/hot zone may not achieve adequate pressure to occlude arterial blood flow. Rapid and bouncy casualty movement to a more secure location may dislodge the tourniquet. Muscle spasms associated with fractured long bones and crepitus may also loosen a tourniquet. Trauma care and fluid resuscitation will raise the patient's blood pressure, resulting in renewed bleeding.

Caregivers need to assess the effectiveness of the tourniquet after every patient movement, as well as during head-to-toe reassessments. There may be a need to add a second tourniquet if the first one is ineffective. A past practice of loosening a tourniquet every 10 to 15 minutes to preserve the limb has been shown to increase hemorrhagic shock with no benefit to the limb. Once a tourniquet is effectively in place it

Table 3-1 Classification of Hemorrhagic Shock

	Class I	Class II	Class III	Class IV
Blood loss (ml)	<750	750–1,500	1,500–2,000	>2,000
Blood loss (% blood volume)	<15%	15–30%	30–40%	>40%
Pulse rate	<100	100–120	120–140	>140
Blood pressure	Normal	Normal	Decreased	Decreased
Pulse pressure (mm Hg)	Normal or increased	Decreased	Decreased	Decreased
Ventilatory rate	14–20	20–30	30–40	>35
Central nervous system/mental status	Slightly anxious	Mildly anxious	Anxious, confused	Confused, lethargic
Fluid replacement	Crystalloid	Crystalloid	Crystalloid and blood	Crystalloid and blood

Note: The values and descriptions for the criteria listed for these classes of shock should not be interpreted as absolute determinants of the class of shock, as significant overlap exists.

Source: From American College of Surgeons (ACS) Committee on Trauma. *Advanced Trauma Life Support for Doctors: Student Course Manual*. 8th ed. Chicago, IL: ACS; 2008.

needs to remain secured. An important note: Never use a training tourniquet operationally. Tourniquets used in field training may become stretched or worn out and are no longer effective on actual casualties.

Venous Tourniquets

A venous tourniquet situation occurs when there is enough pressure to stop venous blood flow but not arterial blood flow. The patient will still have a distal pulse. The extremity will fill with venous blood and swell. This is an ineffective tourniquet, because bleeding from the wound is not controlled. In some situations, the impact of a venous tourniquet may increase hemorrhagic bleeding.

A sign of a venous tourniquet is swelling in the limb. This retention of venous blood in the limb may contribute to the risk of compartment syndrome, which occurs when an extremity is compromised by increased pressure within the limb.

Tourniquet Conversion Contradictions

Conversion is the deliberate process of trying to exchange a tourniquet for a hemostatic agent or a pressure dressing. Tourniquets cause pressure injury to the tissue that is being directly compressed and ischemic injury to the tissue that is no longer perfused. Once the patient is in the evacuation/cold zone a detailed assessment of all wounds and tourniquets is performed. In combat settings, if evacuation to hospital-level definitive care is significantly more than 2 hours, military medics evaluate the use of hemostatic dressings with direct pressure on compressible hemorrhage that does not require a tourniquet.

The military's experience is that there can be complications with the improper application of tourniquets, resulting in venous tourniquets and mechanical damage to tissues. Tourniquets that are applied in the direct threat/hot zone may be applied to wounds that do not actually require tourniquets for definitive hemorrhage control. If the trained medic examines the wound under more secure conditions and determines a tourniquet is not required, he or she should apply an appropriate pressure dressing and release the tourniquet slowly, carefully assessing the extremity for appropriate reperfusion and/or signs of compartment syndrome or vascular compromise.

The following are contraindications for tourniquet conversion:

- The patient can arrive to a hospital-level medical resource within 2 hours.
- The patient exhibits signs of shock.
- Tourniquet is applied to a partial or complete limb amputation.
- Patient has multisystem injuries.

> **CHECK YOUR KNOWLEDGE**
>
> **When is tourniquet conversion indicated?**
>
> a. Evacuation to hospital-level care is more than 2 hours.
> b. Patient exhibits signs of traumatic brain injury.
> c. Patient is hypotensive.
> d. Limb has swollen.

Junctional Hemorrhage

Major vascular injuries within the neck, axilla, and groin (i.e., junctional zones) are not amenable to tourniquet application, and effective pressure dressings are often extremely difficult to apply. The use of improvised explosive devices (IEDS) has increased the military's experience in treating junctional hemorrhage. There has been an increased occurrence of IEDs within civilian settings.

Junctional Tourniquets

Junctional hemorrhage occurs at the junction of an extremity with the torso of the body at an anatomic location that precludes the effective use of an extremity tourniquet to control the bleeding. Junctional hemorrhage includes bleeding from the groin, buttocks, gluteal and pelvic areas, perineum, axilla and shoulder girdle, and the base of the neck.

The lethality of limb injuries is less than at junctional areas, as hemorrhage is slower due to the smaller size of the injured vessels. Junctional hemorrhage also includes extremity bleeding from locations where a tourniquet would not work. Junctional hemorrhage is compressible hemorrhage, which can be controlled in the prehospital environment. The Committee on TCCC recommends three junctional tourniquets, discussed next.

The Combat Ready Clamp

The Combat Ready Clamp (CRoC) is a junctional tourniquet that was designed to exert pressure directly over a wound or indirectly over either the inguinal or axilla junctional areas to occlude the underlying blood vessels and thus stop hemorrhage. It has also been cleared by the U.S. Food and Drug Administration (FDA) for use in control of axillary hemorrhage (**Figure 3-5**).

LESSON 3 Indirect Threat Care/Warm Zone

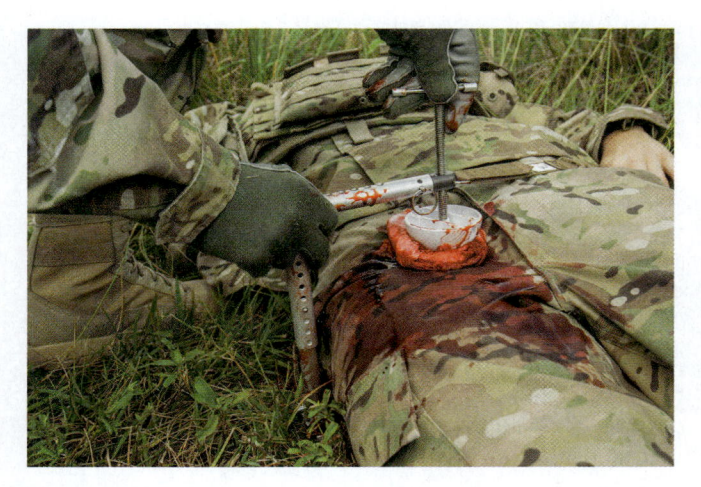

Figure 3-5 The Combat Ready Clamp (CRoC).
Reproduced with permission from Combat Medical. Retrieved from https://combatmedical.com/shop/prod_march/prod_massivehemorrhage/prod_massivehem_croc/

The Junctional Emergency Treatment Tool

The Junctional Emergency Treatment Tool (JETT) incorporates a windlass, much like the Combat Application Tourniquet or Special Operations Forces Tactical Tourniquet, but was designed to compress junctional hemorrhage. The JETT incorporates a pelvic binder application as well as bilateral pads that are designed to occlude femoral artery blood flow to the lower extremities. When used in place of manual pressure, the device frees up healthcare providers to attend to other casualties. JETT components include a belt assembly, two trapezoidal pressure pads, and threaded T-handles. The JETT should not be applied to any casualty for longer than 4 hours (**Figure 3-6**).

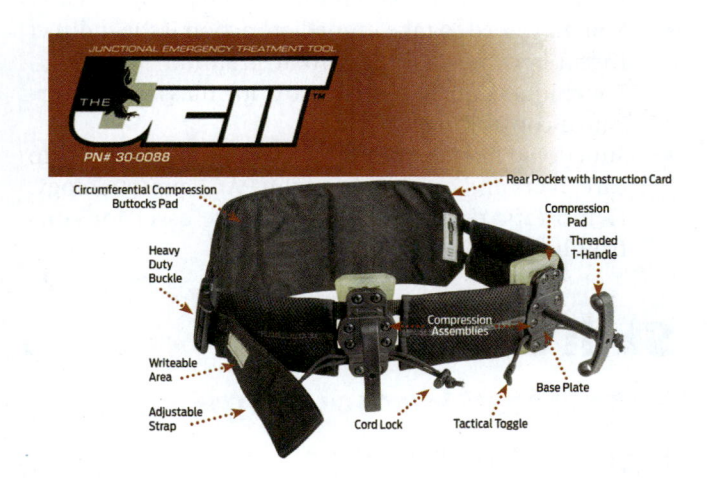

Figure 3-6 Junctional Emergency Treatment Tool (JETT).
Reproduced with permission from North American Rescue. Retrieved from https://www.narescue.com/junctional-emergency-treatment-tool-jett

The SAM Junctional Tourniquet

The SAM Junctional Tourniquet (SJT) is designed to control hemorrhage in areas where bleeding is not amenable to standard tourniquets. Examples include IED or blast injuries or high-level amputations. Components of the SJT include a belt and two pressurized inflatable bladders called target compression devices (TCDs). The TCD is placed at or near the injury site and inflated until the artery is compressed enough to stop the bleeding. If necessary, both TCDs can be used to occlude blood flow bilaterally.

The FDA has cleared the SJT for stabilizing pelvic fractures as well as for controlling junctional bleeding in the axillary area. As with the JETT, application time should not exceed 4 hours (**Figure 3-7**).

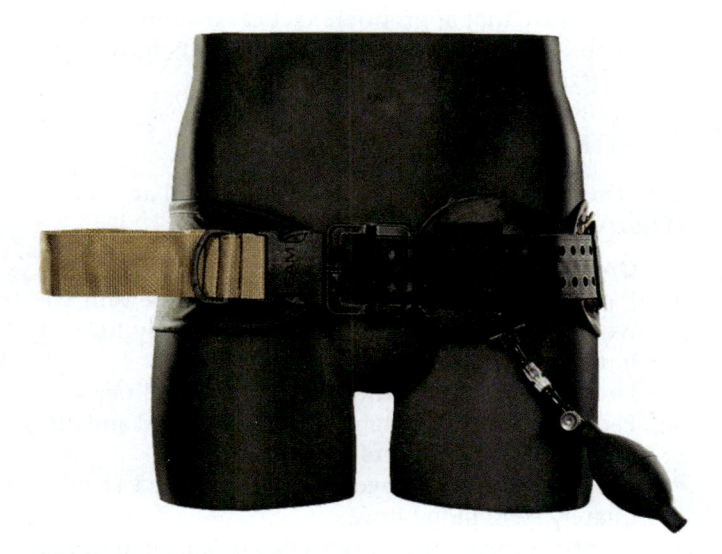

Figure 3-7 SAM Junctional Tourniquet (SJT).
Reproduced with permission from SAM Medical, SAM Junctional Tourniquet. Retrieved from https://www.sammedical.com/products/sam-sjt

Hemostatic Dressings

Hemostatic dressings used by military forces demonstrate successful bleeding control in junctional injuries and any hemorrhage site where a tourniquet cannot be effectively applied. These agents have physical properties that allow them to adhere to damaged tissue and seal ruptured blood vessels or enhance natural blood-clotting mechanisms to accelerate clot formation and produce a strengthened clot.

Clot formation enhancement can be achieved through two mechanisms: (1) concentration of clotting elements in the wound through rapid absorption of water from blood, or (2) chemical reactions that stimulate the intrinsic coagulation pathway. The ideal agent should stop bleeding in 2 minutes or less, cause no toxicity to surrounding tissue, cause no pain or thermal injury, be ready to use with little training, be easily applied under extreme conditions, fit complex wounds, be easily removed from the wound, have a long shelf life, and be cost-effective.

Combat Gauze, a kaolin-impregnated gauze packing agent, is the primary hemostatic agent recommended by the Committee on TCCC. Kaolin is a type of soft white clay that when applied to wounds via packed gauze will activate factor XII, thus accelerating the body's natural clotting ability.

Many TECC units utilize one of two chitosan-based gauze products (Chitogauze and Celox Gauze) with equally successful results. Chitosan is a sugar that is extracted from the shells of crab, lobster, shrimp, and other shellfish. These hemostatic agents are not intended for simple topical application. Therefore, medical directors should ensure that appropriate tactical wound-packing protocols are in place and that practitioners have been properly trained in hemostatic agent use.

Combat Gauze Directions

Use the following steps to apply Combat Gauze (**Figure 3-8**):

- Open clothing around the wound.
- If possible, remove excessive pooled blood from the wound while preserving any clots already formed in the wound.
- Locate the source of the most active bleeding.
- Pack Combat Gauze tightly into the wound and directly onto the source of bleeding.
- Multiple gauze packages may be required to adequately stem blood flow.
- Combat Gauze may be repacked or adjusted in the wound to ensure proper placement.
- Quickly apply pressure until bleeding stops.
- Hold continuous pressure for 3 minutes.
- Reassess to ensure bleeding is controlled.
- Combat Gauze may be repacked or a second gauze used if initial application fails to provide hemostasis.

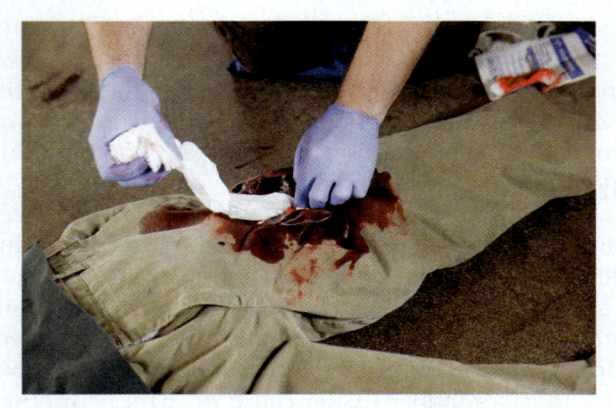

Figure 3-8 Proper packing of wound with Combat Gauze.
© Jones & Bartlett Learning. Photographed by Darren Stahlman.

- Leave Combat Gauze in place.
- Wrap to effectively secure the dressing in the wound.
- Do not remove bandage or Combat Gauze.
- Reassess frequently to monitor for recurrent bleeding.

Some junctional hemorrhages may not be controllable with tourniquets, pressure dressings, or hemostatic agents. If the tactical situation is such that a rescuer cannot maintain prolonged direct manual pressure, a mechanical device, such as one of the junctional tourniquets listed here, may be used to achieve prolonged direct pressure. The C-TECC recommends selecting devices that have been clinically evaluated and have received FDA approval when considering these devices for tactical protocols.

CHECK YOUR KNOWLEDGE

After packing Combat Gauze into a wound and applying pressure until the bleeding stops, you need to hold continuous pressure for at least _____ minutes.

a. 15
b. 10
c. 8
d. 3

Summary

- This lesson has worked through the PACE methodology for a massive hemorrhage progressive and aggressive intervention plan.
- Massive hemorrhage control interventions need to match the dynamic situation and the phases of care.
- You may need to take immediate action if the indirect threat becomes a direct threat situation.
- Tourniquets are the first resort for massive hemorrhage control in extremities.
- Junctional hemorrhage presents unique challenges to caregivers and benefits from the PACE methodology.
- Hemostatic dressings are a valuable asset for controlling junctional hemorrhage.

Skill Stations

Junctional Hemorrhage

Inguinal Hemorrhage

1. Expose the groin area or ensure that the casualty's pockets are empty.
2. Slide the SAM Junctional Tourniquet underneath the casualty.

3. Position the target compression device (TCD) over the femoral pulse point just below the inguinal ligament.
4. Place a hemostatic dressing (or sterile gauze) directly over the wound.
5. Hold the TCD in place and connect the belt by snapping the buckle together.
6. Pull the brown handles away from each other until the buckle secures. You will hear an audible click. Fasten excess belt in place by pressing it down on the Velcro. You may hear a second click once the belt is secure.
7. Use the hand pump to inflate the TCD until hemorrhage stops. In this exercise, the participant will verbalize both inflating the TCD and checking for hemorrhage control.
8. Monitor the casualty during transport for hemorrhage control, and adjust the device if necessary.

Axillary Hemorrhage

1. Prepare the SAM Junctional Tourniquet (SJT) by attaching the extender by pressing the extender onto the brown Velcro.
2. Apply the SJT to the casualty under the arms, as high as possible.
3. On the injured side of the patient, place the D-ring and align with the casualty's neck.
4. Connect the buckle and pull the brown handles apart until you hear a click.
5. Secure the loose end of the strap by pressing down on the Velcro.
6. Attach the large clip on the strap to the D-ring on the front of the SJT.
7. Connect the accessory strap to the cord on the back of the SJT using the small clip, as close as possible to the casualty's midline.
8. Use the hand pump to inflate the TCD until hemorrhage stops. In this exercise, the participant will verbalize both inflating the TCD and checking for hemorrhage control.
9. Monitor the casualty during transport for hemorrhage control, and adjust the device if necessary.

REFERENCES AND RESOURCES

Hodgetts TJ, Mahoney PF, Evans G, Brooks A, editors. *Battlefield Advanced Trauma Life Support*. 3rd ed. Defense Medical Education and Training Agency, Joint Service Publication 570, 2006.

Kotwal RS, Butler FK. Junctional Hemorrhage Control for Tactical Combat Casualty Care. *Wilderness Environ Med.* 2017; 28(2S);S33-S38.

Kotwal RS, Butler FK, Gross KR, Kheirabadi BS, Baer DG, Dubick MA, Rasmussen TE, Weber MA, Bailey JA. Management of junctional hemorrhage in tactical combat casualty care: TCCC guidelines-proposed change 13-03. *J Spec Oper Med.* 2013;13(4):85-93.

National Association of Emergency Medical Technicians. *PHTLS: Prehospital Trauma Life Support*. 9th ed. Burlington, MA: Public Safety Group; 2019.

Pons PT, Jacobs L. SAVE A LIFE: What Everyone Should Know to Stop Bleeding After an Injury. https://www.bleedingcontrol.org/~/media/bleedingcontrol/files/stop%20the%20bleed%20booklet.ashx. American College of Surgeons. 2017. Accessed February 14, 2019.

Shackelford SA, Butler FK Jr, Kragh JF Jr, Stevens RA, Seery JM, Parsons DL, Montgomery HR, Kotwal RS, Mabry RL, Bailey JA. Optimizing the use of limb tourniquets in Tactical Combat Casualty Care: TCCC guidelines change 14-02. *J Spec Oper Med.* 2015; 15(1):17-31.

LESSON 4

Indirect Threat Care/Warm Zone: MARCH—Airway

LESSON OBJECTIVES
- Identify appropriate airway maneuvers for the unconscious versus conscious patient.
- Discuss indications for surgical cricothyrotomy.
- Discuss airway management modifications for pediatric casualties.

Overview of Airway in the Indirect Threat/Warm Zone

Once a casualty's major hemorrhage is controlled, the tactical emergency casualty care (TECC) provider looks to establish and maintain an effective airway. The level of intervention will be based on the patient's level of consciousness, the clinical aspects of airway integrity, and the tactical situation within the indirect threat care/warm zone. If the patient is conscious and able to follow commands, allow the patient to assume a position of comfort. Do not force the patient to lie down.

There should be no attempt at airway intervention if the patient is conscious and breathing adequately. If the patient is unconscious, or conscious but unable to follow commands, caregivers should follow this procedure:

Apply trauma jaw thrust maneuver to open airway.

1. Clear mouth of any foreign bodies (vomit, food, broken teeth, gum, etc.).
2. Consider placing a nasopharyngeal airway.
3. Check for air exchange by listening and feeling for air passing in and out of the airway and looking for bilateral rise and fall of the chest.
4. Place patient in the recovery position to maintain the open airway.
5. If previous measures are unsuccessful and equipment is available under an approved protocol, consider advanced airway interventions:
   a. Supraglottic devices
   b. Oro/nasotracheal intubation
   c. Surgical cricothyrotomy
6. Consider applying oxygen if available.

Trauma Jaw Thrust and Chin Lift Maneuvers

The first effort TECC caregivers should perform to establish a patent airway is to try to open the airway using the trauma jaw thrust maneuver to minimize movement of the head. The cervical spine is maintained in a neutral in-line position. The United Nations Security Officers' Emergency Trauma Bag/Basic First Aid document instructs that the mandible ". . . is thrust forward by placing the thumbs on each zygoma (cheekbone), placing the index and long fingers on the mandible, and at the same angle, pushing the mandible forward."

The trauma chin lift maneuver is used to relieve airway obstructions in patients who are breathing spontaneously. The chin and lower incisors are grasped and then lifted to pull the mandible forward (**Figure 4-1**).

These techniques result in movement of the lower mandible anteriorly (upward) and slightly caudal (toward the feet), pulling the tongue forward, away from the posterior airway, and opening the mouth. The trauma jaw thrust and the trauma chin lift are modifications of the conventional jaw thrust and chin lift. The modifications provide protection to the patient's cervical spine while opening the airway by displacing the tongue from the posterior pharynx. In severe mandibular trauma, attachment of the tongue to the floor of the mouth can be lost, which limits the efficacy of both trauma jaw thrust and trauma chin lift.

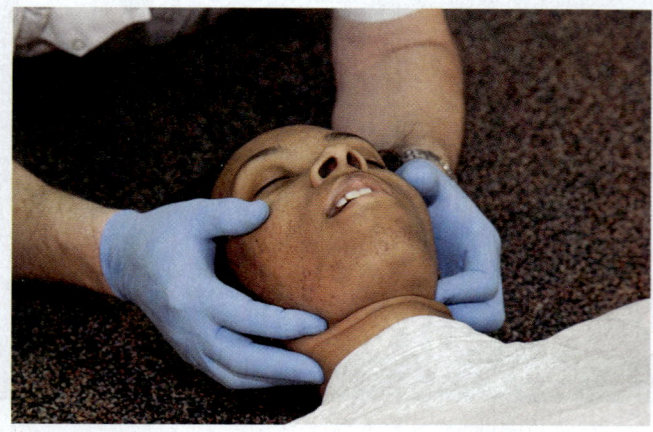

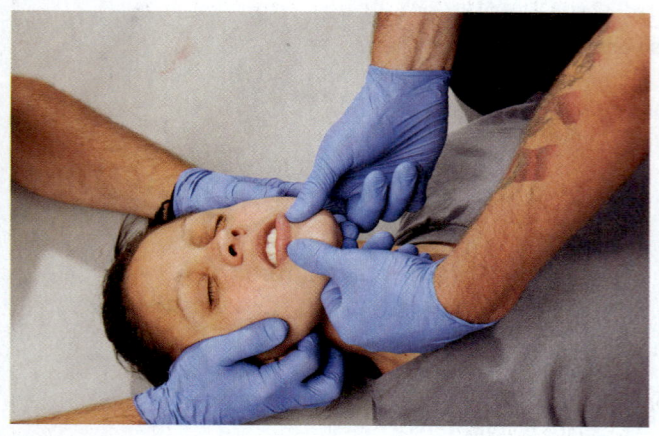

Figure 4-1 **A.** Trauma jaw thrust. The thumb is placed on each zygoma, with the index and long fingers at the angle of the mandible. The mandible is lifted superiorly. **B.** Trauma chin lift. The chin lift performs a function similar to that of the trauma jaw thrust. Moving the mandible forward results in the tongue moving forward to open the airway.

A: © National Association of Emergency Medical Technicians (NAEMT); B: © Jones & Bartlett Learning. Photographed by Darren Stahlman.

After you have opened the patient's airway, look in the patient's mouth to see if anything is blocking the airway. Potential blocks include secretions, such as vomitus, mucus, or blood; foreign objects, such as candy, food, or dirt; and dentures or false teeth that may have become dislodged and are blocking the patient's airway. If you find anything in the patient's mouth, remove it by using a finger sweep. If available in the indirect threat care/warm zone, use suction devices to clear the airway. Remember to check for air exchange by listening and feeling for air passing in and out of the airway and looking for bilateral rise and fall of the chest.

Nasopharyngeal Airway

If spontaneous respirations are present and there is no respiratory distress, an adequate airway may be maintained in an unconscious or unresponsive patient by

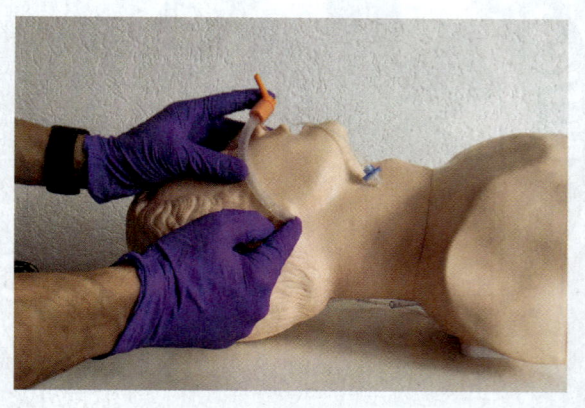

Figure 4-2 Measuring for a nasal airway.
Photograph provided courtesy of J.C. Pitteloud, MD, Switzerland.

the insertion of a nasopharyngeal airway (NPA). This device has the advantage of being better tolerated than an oropharyngeal airway should the patient subsequently regain consciousness and is less likely to be dislodged during patient transport. Evidence has not supported the claim that facial/basilar skull fractures are contraindicated to placement of an NPA.

The NPA is inserted into the patient's nose. You can use nasal airways in both unconscious and conscious patients who are unable to maintain an open airway. An NPA is not as likely to cause vomiting as an oral airway. You will have to select the proper size nasal airway for the patient. Measure from the earlobe to the tip of the patient's nose (**Figure 4-2**).

Coat the NPA with a water-soluble lubricant before inserting it. This step makes it easier for you to insert the device and reduces the chance of causing trauma to the patient's airway. Insert the device in the larger nostril. As you insert the NPA, follow the curvature of the floor of the nose. The NPA is fully inserted when the flange or trumpet rests against the patient's nostril. At this point, the other end of the NPA will reach the back of the patient's throat and it will maintain an open airway for the patient. If available, tape may be used to secure the NPA in place. The procedure to insert an NPA is as follows:

1. Assess the upper airway for visible obstruction.
2. Open the airway with a chin lift/jaw thrust maneuver.
3. Lubricate the NPA with a surgical lubricant.
4. Insert the NPA into the nose at a 90-degree angle to the face. Avoid aiming upward toward the top of the head.
5. Insert all the way to the flange.
6. Use a rotary and/or back-and-forth motion to facilitate insertion.
7. If unable to insert on one side of the nasal passage, take the NPA out and insert on the other side.

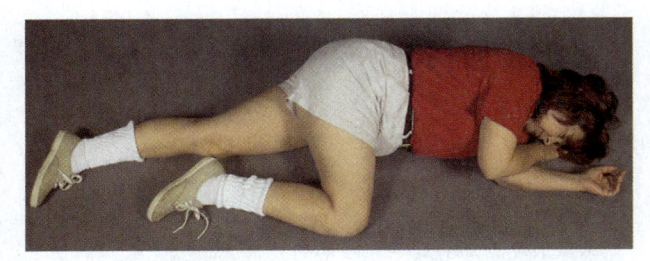

Figure 4-3 Recovery position.
© Jones & Bartlett Learning.

8. Check for air exchange and verify placement of the NPA by listening and feeling for air passing in and out of the airway and looking for bilateral rise and fall of the chest.

Recovery Position

Unconscious patients should be placed in the semi-prone recovery position. This will help prevent patient aspiration of blood, mucus, or vomit (**Figure 4-3**). When positioning the patient on his or her side, stabilize the patient's head and move the entire body in a fluid motion.

The Sit-Up/Lean Forward Position

In a paper reviewing the use of endotracheal intubation, supraglottic airways, and surgical airways, the Committee on Tactical Combat Casualty Care (Co-TCCC) noted "Many casualties with isolated maxillofacial injury can protect their own airways by simply sitting up, leaning forward, spitting out the blood in their airway and continuing to breathe in that position."

Further, the recommendation by the Co-TCCC is that "... surgical airways should be reserved for those casualties in whom (the sit-up/lean forward) strategy is not successful at maintaining an adequate airway." The presence of a maxillofacial injury should not require a surgical airway until the TECC caregiver assesses the status of airway protection with the patient in the sit-up/lean forward position. A surgical airway is the airway procedure of choice when the airway is compromised by direct maxillofacial trauma.

CHECK YOUR KNOWLEDGE

Which of these is the easiest and most effective technique to maintain an airway for an unresponsive patient under tactical conditions?

a. Surgical airway
b. Endotracheal intubation
c. Oropharyngeal airway
d. Nasopharyngeal airway

Complex Airways

Complex airway adjuncts and management techniques are appropriate when simple airway maneuvers and devices are inadequate to maintain a patent airway. Anytime a complex airway device is considered for placement in a patient, the TECC provider must consider the possibility that the procedure will be unsuccessful and have a backup plan in mind. Alternate methods of managing the airway should be considered and the necessary equipment prepared in the event the first choice of intervention proves unsuccessful.

Remember that operators in the indirect threat care/warm zone may need to quickly move if the situation deteriorates. For TECC, complex airway adjuncts include supraglottic devices, orotracheal intubation, nasotracheal intubation, and surgical cricothyrotomy.

Supraglottic Airways

Supraglottic airways offer a functional alternative airway to endotracheal intubation (**Figure 4-4**).

These devices are inserted without direct visualization of the vocal cords. They are also a useful backup airway when endotracheal intubation attempts are unsuccessful, or when, after careful evaluation of the airway, the prehospital care provider feels that the chance for successful placement is higher than for endotracheal intubation.

A supraglottic airway is the primary airway device for an unconscious trauma patient who lacks a gag reflex and is apneic or breathing at a rate of less than 10 breaths/minute. In addition to the supraglottic airway, the patient may need to be ventilated using a bag-mask device or ventilator. For advanced life support (ALS)-credentialed TECC caregivers, the supraglottic airway is often the alternative airway device

SPOTLIGHT

Supraglottic Airway Contraindications and Complications

Contraindications
- Intact gag reflex
- Known esophageal disease
- Recent ingestion of caustic substances

Complications
- Gagging and vomiting (if gag reflex is intact)
- Aspiration
- Damage to the esophagus
- Hypoxia if ventilated using the incorrect lumen

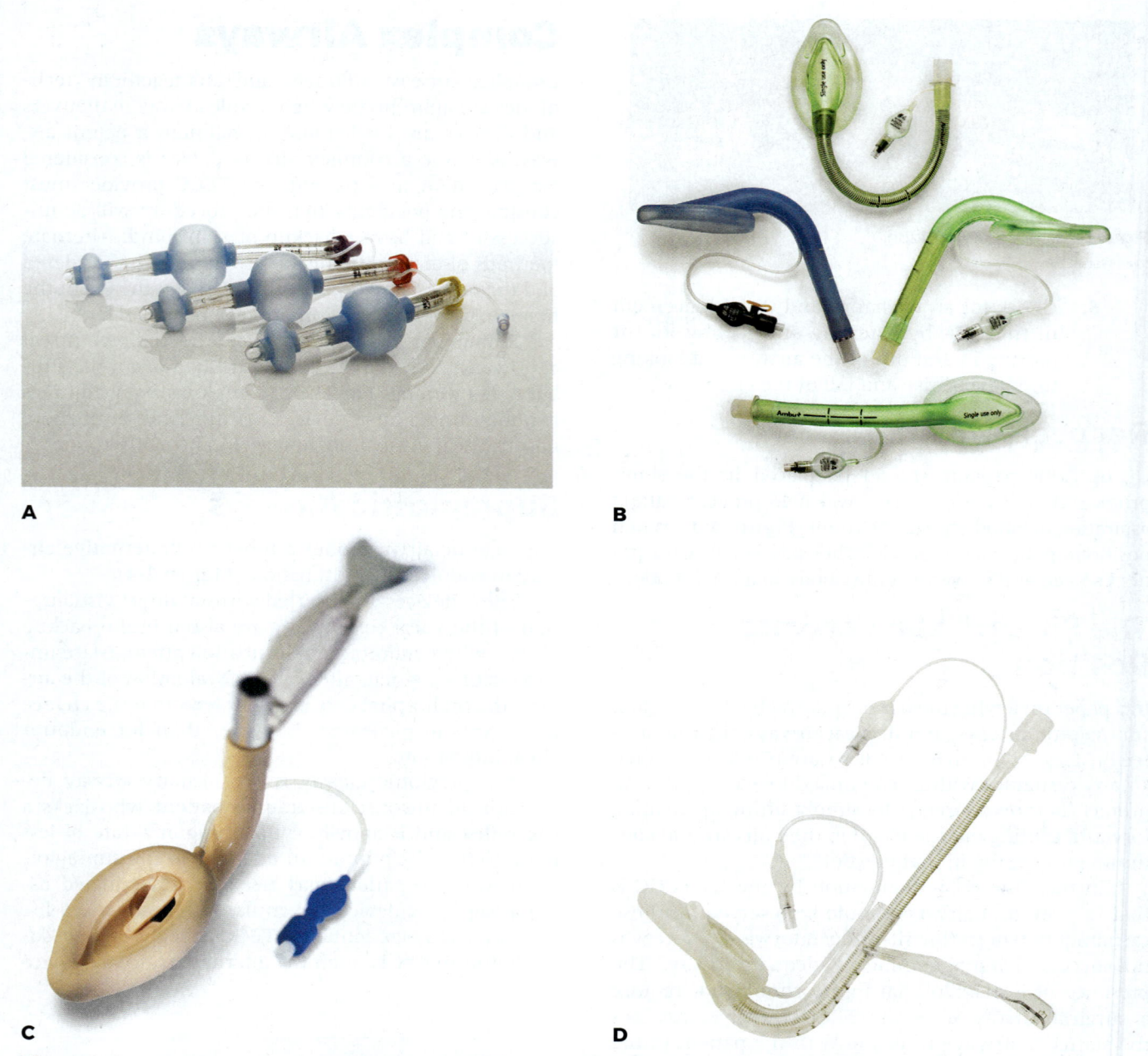

Figure 4-4 **A.** King laryngotracheal airway. **B.** Laryngeal mask airway (LMA). **C.** Intubating LMA. **D.** Intubating LMA with endotracheal tube in place.
A & B: Courtesy of Ambu, Inc; **C & D:** Courtesy of Teleflex, Inc.

when he or she is unable to perform endotracheal intubation and cannot easily ventilate the patient with a bag-mask device with a NPA.

The primary advantage of supraglottic airway devices is that they may be inserted independent of the patient's position and can be performed under poor lighting conditions, both of which may be especially important in trauma patients with access and extrication difficulties or a high suspicion of cervical injury.

When placed into a patient, supraglottic airway devices are designed to isolate the trachea from the esophagus. None of these devices provides a complete seal of the trachea; therefore, while the risk of aspiration is lowered, it is not completely prevented. The procedure to insert a supraglottic airway is described as follows:

1. Check/prepare the supraglottic airway device.
2. Lubricate the distal tip of the device.
3. Position head properly.
4. Perform a tongue-jaw lift.
5. Insert device to proper depth.
6. Secure device in patient.

7. Ventilate patient with bag-mask device and confirm proper ventilation (correct lumen and proper insertion depth) by auscultation bilaterally over lungs and over epigastrium.
8. Adjust ventilation as necessary.
9. Verify proper tube placement by secondary confirmation, if available.
10. Secure the device or confirm that the device remains properly secured.
11. Ventilate the patient at proper rate and volume.

Some manufacturers have developed supraglottic airways in pediatric sizes. Ensure proper sizing according to the manufacturer's specifications if using these types of airways on pediatric patients.

Orotracheal and Nasotracheal Intubation

Orotracheal intubation involves placing an endotracheal (ET) tube into the trachea through the mouth. The non-trauma patient is often placed in a "sniffing" position to facilitate intubation. Because this position hyperextends the cervical spine at C1-C2, the second most common site for cervical spine fractures in the trauma patient, and hyperflexes it at C5-C6, the most common site for cervical spine fractures in the trauma patient, it should not be used for patients with blunt trauma (**Figure 4-5**).

In conscious trauma patients or in those with an intact gag reflex, endotracheal intubation may be difficult to accomplish. If spontaneous ventilations are present, blind nasotracheal intubation (BNTI) may be attempted if the benefit outweighs the risk. Although nasotracheal intubation is often more difficult to perform than direct visualization and oral intubation, a 90% success rate has been reported in trauma patients. During BNTI, the patient must be breathing to ensure that the ET tube is passed through the vocal cords. Many texts suggest that BNTI is contraindicated in the presence of mid-face trauma or fractures, but an exhaustive literature search reveals no documentation of an ET tube entering the cranial vault. Apnea is a contraindication specific to BNTI. In addition, no stylet is used when BNTI is performed.

Face-to-face intubation is indicated when standard trauma intubation techniques cannot be used because of the inability of the prehospital care provider to assume the standard position at the head of the trauma patient. Vehicle entrapment or a patient pinned in rubble are situations that may require face-to-face intubation.

> **CHECK YOUR KNOWLEDGE**
>
> **A bag-mask device is required when using a(n) _____ to maintain an airway.**
>
> a. oropharyngeal airway
> b. supraglottic airway
> c. nasopharyngeal airway
> d. esophageal shunt

Surgical Cricothyrotomy

When direct control of the airway is not possible by other methods, a cricothyrotomy is performed by a TECC caregiver. This is an in-field surgical procedure in which an opening is made through the cricothyroid membrane to allow the placement of a tracheal tube into the neck (**Figure 4-6**).

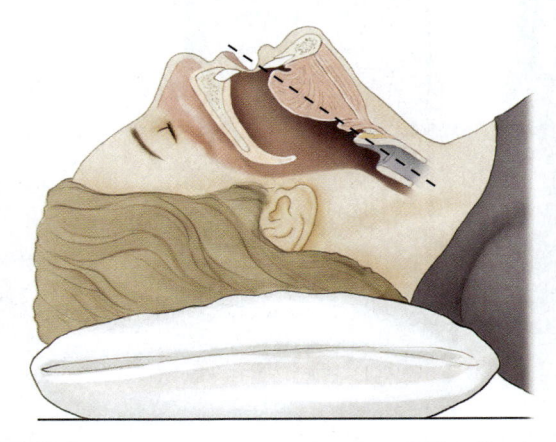

Figure 4-5 Placing the patient's head in the "sniffing" position provides ideal visualization of the larynx through the mouth; however, such positioning hyperextends the patient's neck at C1 and C2 and hyperflexes it at C5 and C6. These are the two most common points of fracture of the cervical spine.

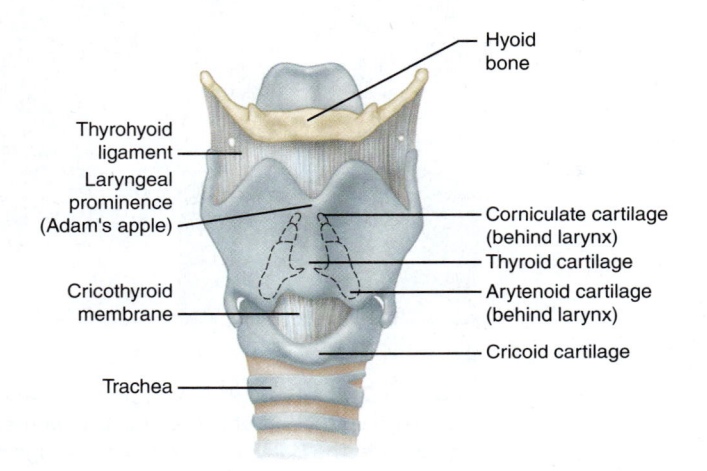

Figure 4-6 Structures involved in a cricothyrotomy.

Surgical cricothyrotomy has been reported to be safe and effective in trauma victim care. For ALS-credentialed TECC caregivers working in the indirect threat care/warm zone, surgical cricothyrotomy may be appropriate to consider as the next step when a NPA is not effective. According to *Conflict and Catastrophe Medicine: A Practical Guide*, cricothyrotomy ". . . may be the only feasible alternative in cases of maxillofacial wounds in which blood or disrupted anatomy precludes visualization of the vocal cords and the sit-up/lean forward position is ineffective in maintaining a secure airway."

Many vendors provide emergency surgical cricothyrotomy kits, which include the following items:

- Endotracheal (ET) tube, sized between 6.0 and 7.0 millimeters (mm)
- ET tube holder
- Curved Kelly hemostats or a tracheal hook to enhance the boundaries of the incision
- Tracheal dilator
- Syringe with a Luer lock tip
- Personal protective equipment (PPE) face shield with ear loop
- Disposable scalpel
- Antiseptic
- Gauze, 4 × 4 inch

Depending on the tactical situation and available resources, a bag-mask device and oxygen source would be beneficial in the indirect threat/warm zone. These items should be available in the cold zone.

Cricothyrotomy Surface Landmarks

The cricothyroid membrane is the tissue between the cricoid and the thyroid cartilage. A cricothyrotomy is the surgical placement of a tube through the cricothyroid membrane. With a patient lying supine and the head in a neutral midline position, palpate the thyroid cartilage, also known as the Adam's apple. The Difficult Airway Society 2015 guidelines describe the "laryngeal handshake" to identify the structures (**Figure 4-7**). The Difficult Airway Society recommends use of the laryngeal handshake ". . . as the first step because it promotes confidence in the recognition of the three-dimensional anatomy of the laryngeal structures; the conical cartilaginous cage consisting of the hyoid, thyroid, and cricoid. The laryngeal handshake is performed with the nondominant hand, identifying the hyoid and thyroid laminae, stabilizing the larynx between thumb and middle finger, and moving down the neck to palpate the cricothyroid membrane with the index finger."

Using a buddy, the TECC student should be able to demonstrate the following landmarks used to locate the cricothyroid membrane (**Figure 4-8**):

- Top of the thyroid cartilage
- Thyroid prominence (Adam's apple); usually visible in males
- Bottom of thyroid cartilage
- Cricothyroid membrane
- Cricoid cartilage

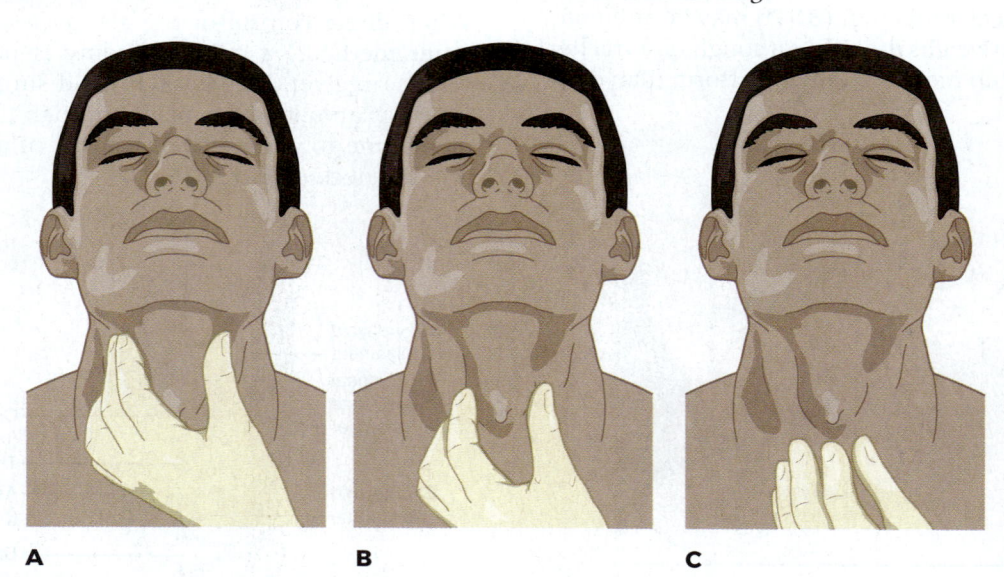

Figure 4-7 The Difficult Airway Society's laryngeal handshake. **A.** The index finger and thumb grasp the top of the larynx (the greater cornu of the hyoid bone) and roll it from side to side. The bony and cartilaginous cage of the larynx is a cone, which connects to the trachea. **B.** The fingers and thumb slide down over the thyroid laminae. **C.** Middle finger and thumb rest on the cricoid cartilage, with the index finger palpating the cricothyroid membrane.

C. Frerk, et. al. Difficult Airway Society 2015 guidelines for management of unanticipated difficult intubation in adults, Oxford University Press, 2015.

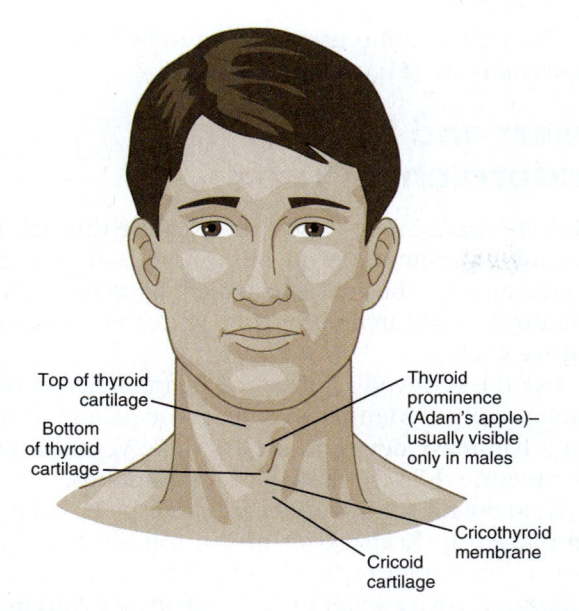

Figure 4-8 Surface landmarks for cricothyrotomy (exterior view).
© Jones & Bartlett Learning.

The cricothyroid membrane is the best location to establish a surgical emergency airway. This is a small gap, with the thyroid cartilage above the gap and the anterior cricoid ring below the gap. The thyroid gland is attached to the side of the thyroid cartilage, with four great vessels below the gland. In a 2015 article in *EMS Word*, Collopy notes that ". . . these blood vessels increase the risk of bleeding during procedures in this anatomic region and thus the region is best avoided."

The cricothyroid membrane is a small space, with an average vertical width of 9 mm and an average horizontal length of 30 mm. This space is large enough to accept a 6.0-mm endotracheal airway, which has an outer diameter of 8.2 mm. It would be a challenge for most patients to accept an 8.0-mm ET tube as it has an 11.0-mm outer diameter. Better to have a smaller, secured airway than trying to force a larger tube through the cricothyroid membrane (**Figure 4-9**).

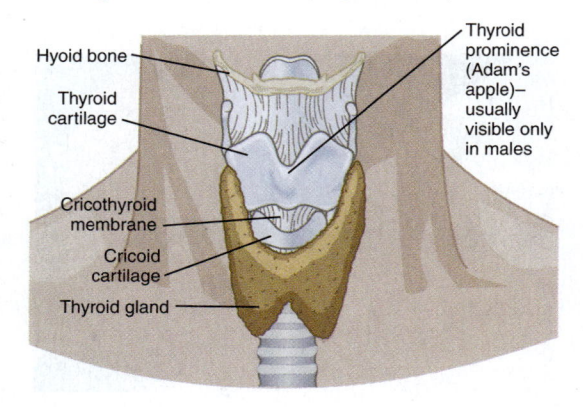

Figure 4-9 Surface landmarks for cricothyrotomy (interior view).
© Jones & Bartlett Learning.

> ## SPOTLIGHT
> **TECC Emergency Surgical Airway Steps**
> 1. Assemble and test all the necessary equipment.
> 2. Assess the upper airway for visible obstruction.
> 3. Identify the cricothyroid membrane between the thyroid and cricoid cartilages. Identify the location of the top of the thyroid cartilage, the thyroid prominence (on males), the bottom of the thyroid cartilage, the top of the cricoid cartilage, and the cricothyroid membrane.
> 4. Identify the site of the skin incision.
> 5. Palpate the cricothyroid membrane and (while stabilizing the cartilage) make a vertical incision through skin directly over the cricothyroid membrane.
> 6. While continuing to stabilize the larynx, use the scalpel or a hemostat to cut or poke through the cricothyroid membrane.
> 7. Insert the tips of the hemostat through the opening and open the jaws to dilate the opening. A tracheal hook may also be used for this purpose, but care should be exercised as these hooks place the ET/trach balloon at risk.
> 8. Insert the ET tube between the jaws of the hemostat; the tube should be in the trachea and directed toward the lungs.
> 9. Inflate the cuff.
> 10. Check for air exchange and verify placement of the tube by **listening and feeling for air passing in and out of the tube, causing the tube to mist, and looking for bilateral rise and fall of the chest.**
> 11. If the position is correct, secure the tube with tape or a commercial tube-securing device.
> 12. Apply a dressing to further protect the tube and incision site.
> 13. Monitor the casualty's respirations. Ventilate if required.

Cricothyrotomy Incision

The recommended field emergency technique is to make a vertical incision through the skin and a horizontal incision through the cricothyroid membrane. If further exposure is needed, the incision can be extended at either end.

Once the opening is made, use a dilator or tool to enlarge or maintain the opening. The TECC caregiver can use a finger, tracheal hook, curved forceps, or scalpel handle to enlarge or maintain the opening. Finally, the ET or tracheostomy tube is inserted.

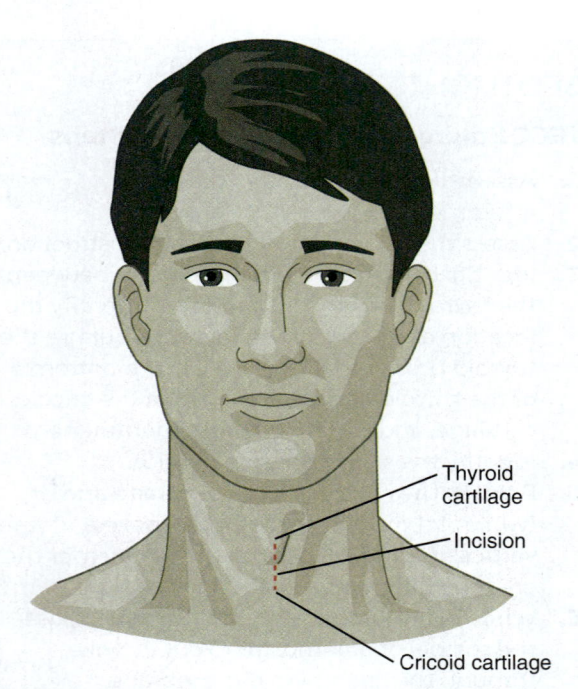

Figure 4-10 Locating the cricothyroid incision line.
© Jones & Bartlett Learning.

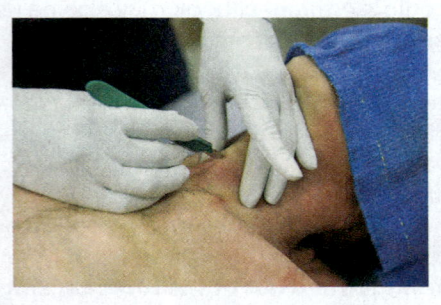

Figure 4-11 Expose the cricothyroid membrane.
© Jones & Bartlett Learning.

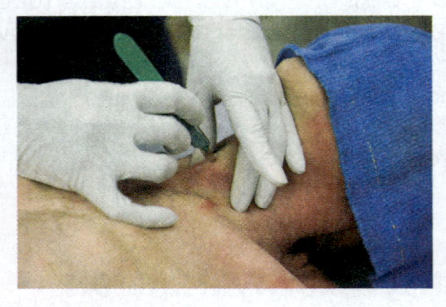

Figure 4-12 Make a single stabbing incision through the cricothyroid membrane.
© Jones & Bartlett Learning.

Start the incision with the scalpel (**Figure 4-10**). Carefully cut through and expand the skin layers to the point that you have exposed the cricothyroid membrane (**Figure 4-11**).

Make a single stabbing incision through the cricothyroid membrane with the scalpel (**Figure 4-12**).

Open the incision using curved Kelly hemostats or a tracheal hook (**Figure 4-13**).

Insert and Secure Endotracheal Tube

Lubricate the ET tube. Insert the ET tube through the cricothyroid membrane no more than 3 to 4 inches into the airway. The goal is to avoid having the ET tube slip into the right main bronchus with any movement (**Figure 4-14**).

Use the syringe to inflate the endotracheal airway balloon with air. Manually ventilate the patient or connect a bag-mask device to the ET tube. Ventilate with two breaths while checking for breath sounds.

If no breath sounds are heard, pull the ET tube out and reinsert it. Recheck for breath sounds to confirm that the tube is correctly placed. If available, connect a bag-mask device to an oxygen supply. As with every advanced airway, this should be double checked with ETCO$_2$ if available. Secure the tube and cover the opening with gauze dressing (**Figure 4-15**).

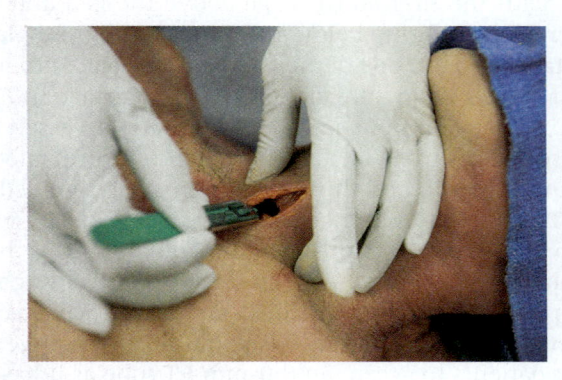

Figure 4-13 Open the incision.
© Jones & Bartlett Learning.

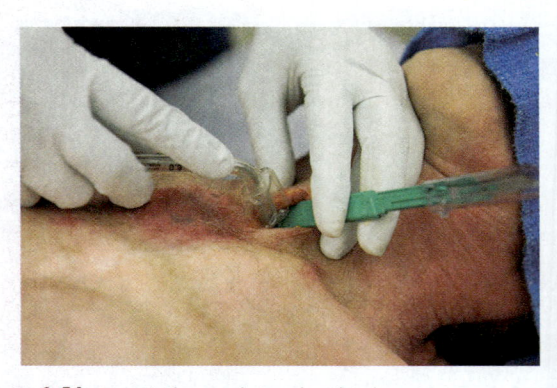

Figure 4-14 Insert the endotracheal tube.
© Jones & Bartlett Learning.

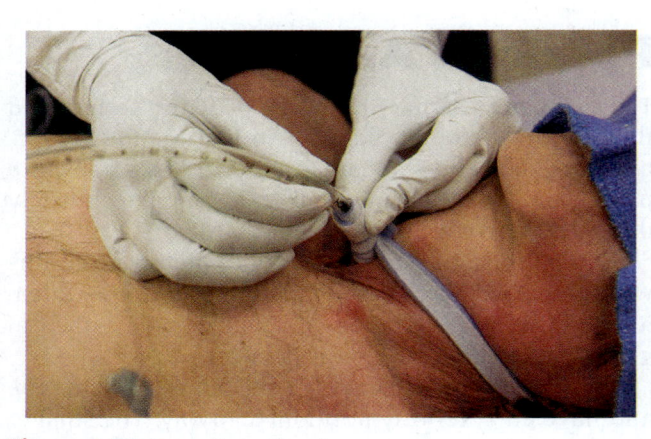

LESSON 4 Indirect Threat Care/Warm Zone: MARCH—Airway

Figure 4-15 Dress the wound.
© Jones & Bartlett Learning.

Bougie-Assisted Placement of ET Tube in Surgical Airway

The bougie-assisted emergency cricothyrotomy technique (BACT) is a modification of the rapid four-step technique (RFST) using a bougie to guide insertion of the ET tube. The four steps in RFST are: (1) palpation, (2) stab incision, (3) inferior traction, and (4) tube insertion. This streamlined method is simple and quick. Because the operator's body position and hand movements (steps 3 and 4) are similar to those in orotracheal intubation, there is a feeling of familiarity that enhances retention of the procedure.

The BACT uses the least amount of equipment and has shown better effectiveness on the battleground than other procedures.

1. Use the scalpel to incise neck tissue.
2. Use caregiver's fingers to move neck tissue to expose the cricothyroid membrane.
3. Stabilize the trachea using the thumb and middle finger of the nondominant hand.
4. Confirm cricothyroid membrane location.
5. Make a transverse incision with the scalpel.
6. Apply tracheal hook to secure trachea to incision opening (**Figure 4-16**).
7. Insert bougie through trachea.
8. Insert 6.0-mm ET tube over the bougie and into incision opening.
9. Inflate tracheal lumen.
10. Remove bougie.

The procedure demonstrated during the TECC course shows the bougie used to hold the trachea in place after the stab incision is completed.

While maintaining the opening with the tracheal hook, carefully insert the flexible end of the bougie into the opening and down the trachea (**Figure 4-17**). Do not lacerate the trachea with the bougie.

While advancing the bougie, feel for the "bump" as the tip of the bougie advances down the trachea and touches the tracheal rings. Once the bougie is past the patient's sternal notch, insert the ET tube on the bougie and advance the tube through the incision (**Figure 4-18**).

Once the tube is in place, inflate the lumen and remove the bougie and tracheal hook (**Figure 4-19**).

Ventilate and confirm placement of the ET tube by looking for chest rise or misting within the tube, listening for lung sounds, or observing changes in capnography color or $ETCO_2$.

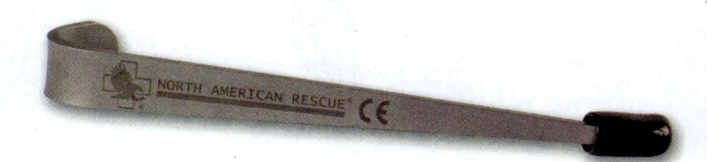

Figure 4-16 Tracheal hook.
Reproduced with permission from North American Rescue. Retrieved from https://www.narescue.com/nar-tracheal-hook

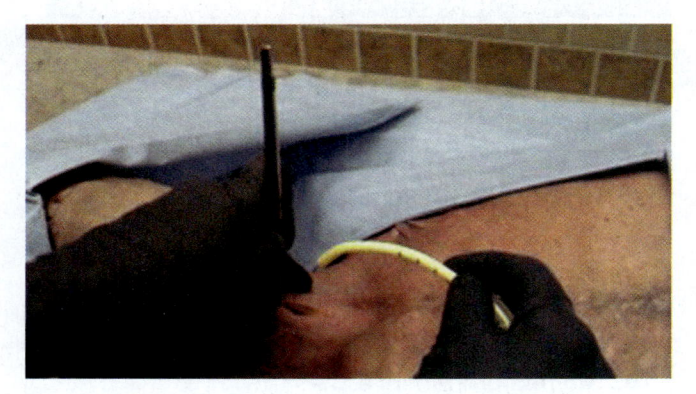

Figure 4-17 Control the trachea and insert the bougie.
Courtesy of Centre for Emergency Health Sciences.

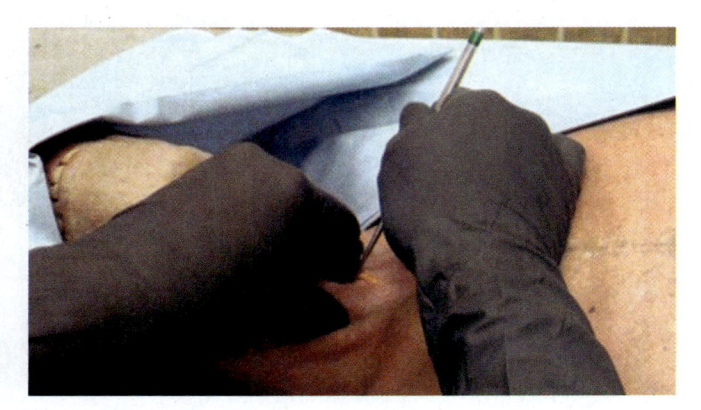

Figure 4-18 Insert the ET tube.
Courtesy of Centre for Emergency Health Sciences.

A

B

Figure 4-19 Stabilize the tube.
Courtesy of Centre for Emergency Health Sciences.

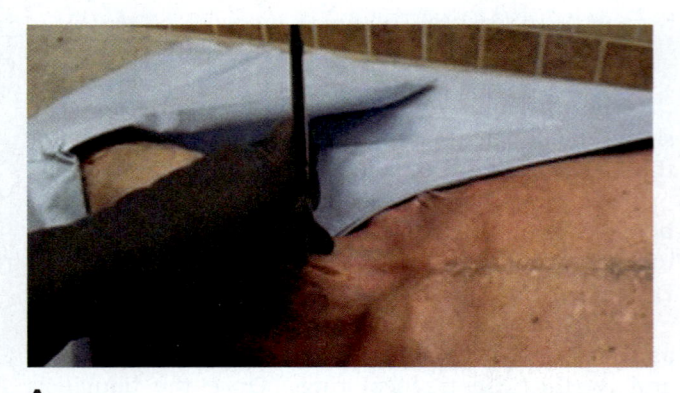

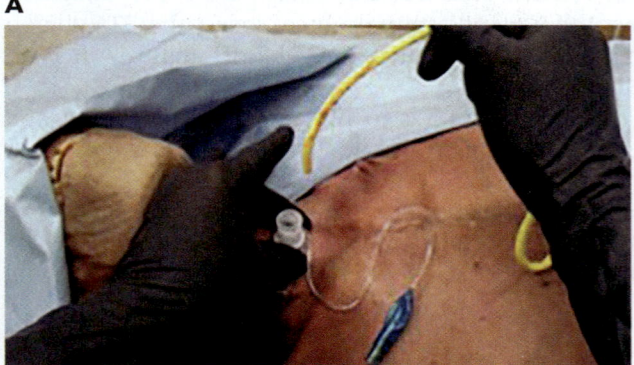

CHECK YOUR KNOWLEDGE

A cricothyrotomy incision is made to the:

a. cricoid cartilage.
b. thyroid cartilage.
c. cricothyroid membrane.
d. thyroid prominence.

Pediatric Airways

The small and variable size of the pediatric patient and the unique anatomic characteristics of the airway frequently make the standard procedures to establish a patent airway in a child challenging and technically difficult (**Figure 4-20**).

Attempting to place an inappropriately sized airway can do more harm than good. Color-coded, length-based resuscitation guides provide practical medication and equipment references.

Children have a relatively large occiput and tongue and have an anteriorly positioned airway. The smaller the child, the greater the size discrepancy between the cranium and the midface. Therefore, the relatively large occiput forces passive flexion of the cervical spine (**Figure 4-21**).

These factors all predispose children to a higher risk of anatomic airway obstruction than adults. A patent airway should be ensured and maintained with suctioning, manual maneuvers, and airway adjuncts. Initial management in the pediatric patient includes in-line cervical spine stabilization. Unless a specialized pediatric spine board that has a depression at the head is used, adequate padding (2 to 3 centimeters [about 1 inch]) should be placed under the torso of the small child so that the cervical spine is maintained in a straight line rather than forced into slight flexion because of the disproportionately large occiput. When adjusting and maintaining airway positioning, compressing the soft tissues of the neck and trachea should be avoided (**Figure 4-22**).

Pediatric Nasopharyngeal Airway

Consider using a pediatric NPA for the unconscious or conscious and unresponsive child without an airway

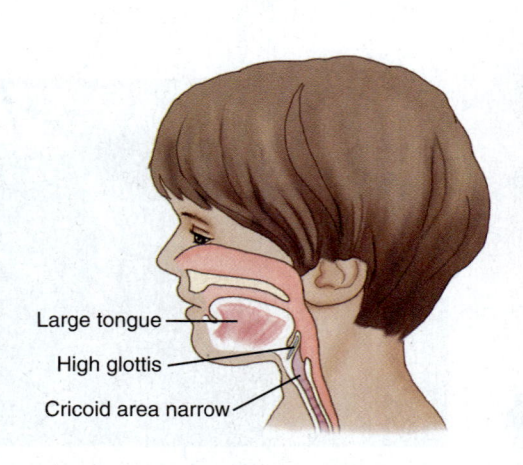

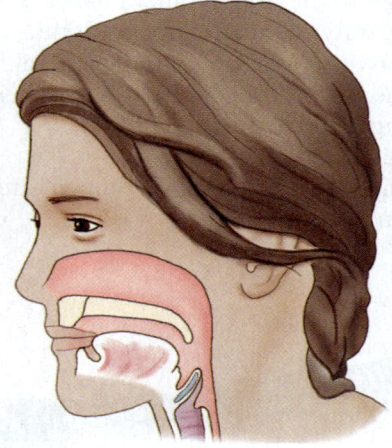

- Large tongue
- High glottis
- Cricoid area narrow

Figure 4-20 Comparison of the adult and child airways.
© National Association of Emergency Medical Technicians (NAEMT).

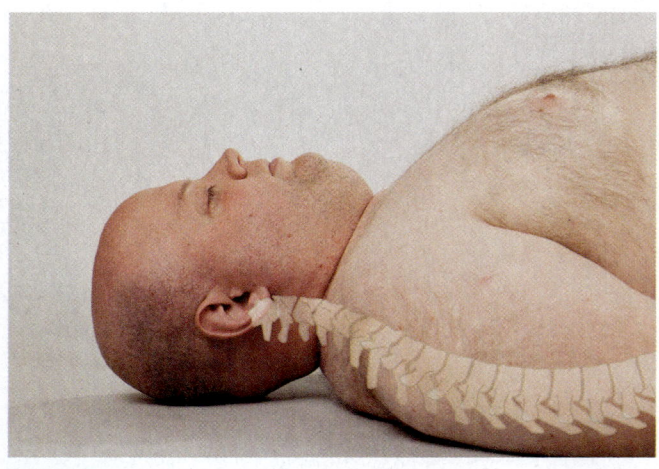

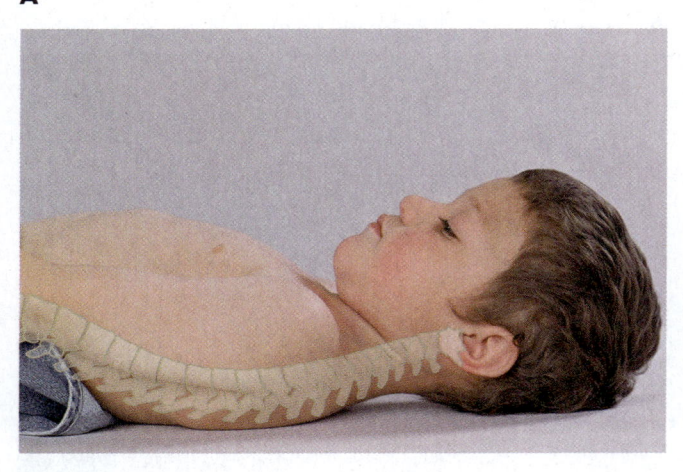

obstruction. The procedure to use a pediatric NPA is similar to an adult.

1. Determine the appropriate size NPA. The external diameter of the NPA should not be larger than the diameter of the nares, and there should be no blanching of the nares after insertion.
2. Place the NPA next to the pediatric patient's face to make sure the length is correct. The NPA should extend from the tip of the nose to the tragus of the ear. The tragus is the small cartilaginous projection in front of the opening of the ear.
3. Position the pediatric patient's airway, using the techniques described earlier for the oropharyngeal airway.
4. Lubricate the NPA with a water-soluble lubricant.
5. Insert the tip into the right naris (nostril opening) with the bevel pointing toward the septum, or central divider in the nose. The right naris is commonly larger than the left naris in most patients.
6. Carefully move the tip forward, following the roof of the mouth, until the flange rests against the outside of the nostril. If you are inserting the NPA on the left side, insert the tip into the left naris upside down, with the bevel pointing toward the septum. Move the NPA forward slowly about 1" until you feel a slight resistance, and then rotate the airway 180°.
7. Reassess the NPA after insertion.

Reproduced with permission from the American Academy of Orthopaedic Surgeons, Emergency Care and Transportation of the Sick and Injured, Eleventh Edition, pages 1247–1249

A NPA with a small diameter may easily become obstructed by mucus, blood, vomitus, or the soft tissues of the pharynx. If the NPA is too long, it may stimulate the vagus nerve and slow the heart rate or enter the esophagus, causing gastric distention. Inserting the NPA in responsive patients may cause a spasm of the larynx and result in vomiting. NPAs should not be used in patients under 1 year of age and when patients have facial trauma because the NPA may tear soft tissues and cause bleeding into the airway. Depending on the injuries, consider placing the patient in the recovery position.

Pediatric Supraglottic Airway

Authors Jagannathan, Ramsey, White, and Sohn note that ". . . supraglottic airways facilitate oxygenation and ventilation while sitting immediately outside the larynx to form a perilaryngeal seal. [Supraglottic airways] are an established part of routine and emergency pediatric airway management, including use in the difficult airway and neonatal resuscitation." They come in a variety of sizes.

Figure 4-21 Compared to an adult **(A)**, a child has a larger occiput and less shoulder musculature. When placed on a flat surface, these factors result in flexion of the neck **(B)**.
A & B: © National Association of Emergency Medical Technicians (NAEMT).

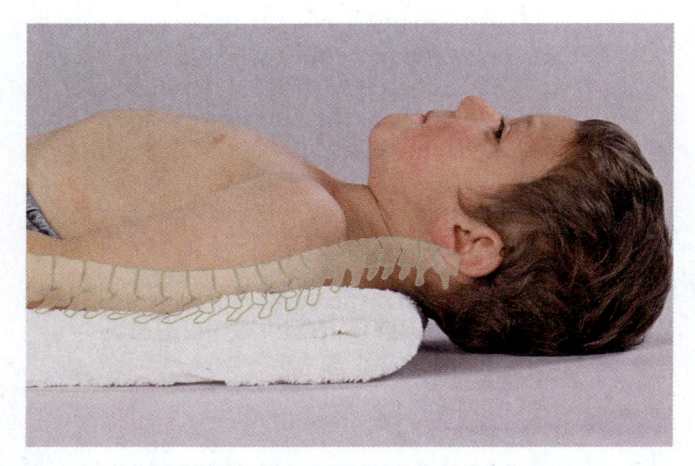

Figure 4-22 Provide adequate padding under the child's torso or use a spine board with a cutout for the child's occiput.
© National Association of Emergency Medical Technicians (NAEMT).

Further, Jagannathan et al. state, "Supraglottic airways may be classified as first- or second-generation devices based on the presence of a gastric access channel. First-generation devices are simple airway tubes attached to a mask that rests over the glottic opening. Second-generation devices incorporate a gastric access channel that allows for gastric venting, and the option to place a gastric tube." When placed correctly, the supraglottic airway provides two seals within the patent airway.

If available, apply oxygen. In the out-of-hospital environment, using a bag-mask device with a supraglottic airway device is the equivalent in effectiveness to an intubated adult with a bag-mask device.

Advanced Pediatric Airways

Pediatric intubation is an advanced airway option that may be difficult to perform within the indirect threat care/warm zone due to the dynamic conditions at the incident scene, limited supplies, and the risk/reward in completing the procedure, especially if there is an imminent evacuation time or a short transport to the evacuation zone.

If confronted with a "cannot ventilate" situation after using a supraglottic airway, a surgical airway may be the more appropriate response. The pediatric cricothyroid membrane is much smaller and more difficult to palpate. A percutaneous needle cricothyrotomy is recommended as it presents less risk of injury to vital structures.

The recommended technique is:

1. Position the child so that the neck is extended and the trachea and larynx are forced forward (if there is no cervical spine injury), e.g., with a folded blanket or towel roll.
2. Palpate the center of the thyroid cartilage, and with the fingernail move toward the toes until the indentation of the cricothyroid membrane is located.
3. Puncture the cricothyroid membrane in a downward direction using a large-bore intravenous catheter with syringe attached and aspirate for air to confirm intratracheal position; if air cannot be aspirated then the catheter needle tip is misplaced and this step is repeated (**Figure 4-23A**).
4. After aspiration of air, advance the catheter off the needle into the trachea, withdraw the needle and syringe, and again attach the syringe to the catheter.
5. Again aspirate for air to reconfirm continued intratracheal position.
6. Attach the catheter to the adapter of a 3.0-mm internal diameter ET tube, which then allows connection with any standard bag-mask device. Alternatively, attach the barrel of a 3-ml syringe to the IV catheter and place an 8.0-mm internal diameter ET tube adapter in the barrel of the syringe (**Figure 4-23B**).

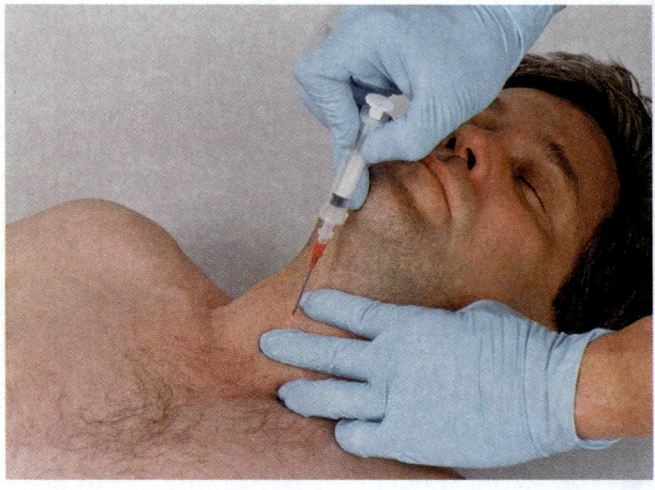

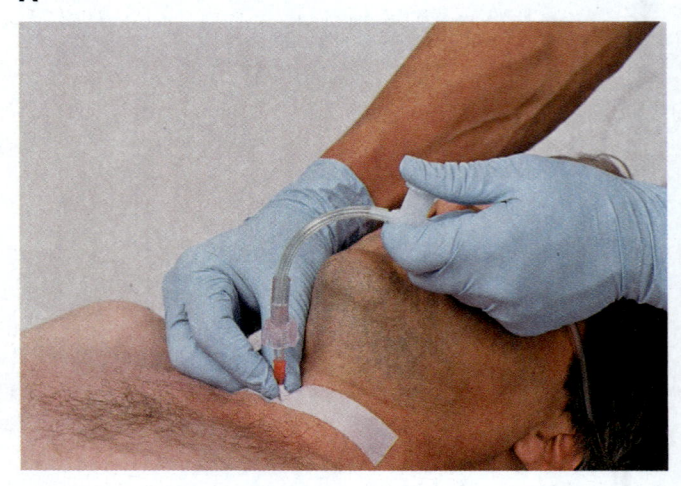

Figure 4-23 Percutaneous needle cricothyrotomy.
A & B: © National Association of Emergency Medical Technicians (NAEMT).

CHECK YOUR KNOWLEDGE

Which of these is an important anatomic difference to consider with airway control in a pediatric patient?

a. Larger tongue
b. Lower tidal volume
c. Reduced size discrepancy between the cranium and midface
d. Posterior positioned airway

Summary

- If the casualty is conscious, let the patient sit up and lean forward.
- If the casualty is unconscious, the first-line option is a trauma jaw thrust followed by an NPA.
- Consider cricothyrotomy as the first-line airway procedure for maxillofacial trauma with airway obstruction or inhalation burns.
- Do not place pediatric patients in a supine position without supporting the neck and back.
- Position the airway according to the pediatric casualty's size.

Skill Stations

Nasopharyngeal Airway

1. Assemble and test all necessary equipment.
2. Assess the upper airway for visible obstruction.
3. Open the airway with a chin lift–jaw thrust maneuver.
4. Identify the indications for an NPA (unconscious patient).
5. Lubricate the NPA with a surgical lubricant.
6. Insert the airway into the nose at a 90-degree angle to the face. Avoid aiming upward toward the top of the head. Insert all the way to the flange.
7. Use a rotary and/or back-and-forth motion to facilitate insertion.
8. If unable to insert the airway on one side of the nasal passage, take it out and try the other side.

Supraglottic Airway

1. Open the airway manually.
2. Elevate the tongue, and insert simple adjunct.
3. Ventilate patient with bag-mask device unattached to oxygen.
4. Attach oxygen reservoir to bag-mask device and connect to high-flow oxygen regulator (12–15 l/min).
5. Ventilate patient at a rate of 10 to 12 breaths/min with appropriate volumes.
6. Direct assistant to preoxygenate patient.
7. Check/prepare supraglottic airway device.
8. Lubricate distal tip of the device (may be verbalized).
9. Position head properly.
10. Perform a tongue-jaw lift.
11. Insert device to proper depth.
12. Secure device in patient.
13. Ventilate patient and confirm proper ventilation (correct lumen and proper insertion depth) by auscultation bilaterally over lungs and over epigastrium.
14. Adjust ventilation as necessary.
15. Verify proper tube placement by secondary confirmation such as capnography, capnometry, esophageal detector device, or colorimetric device.
16. Secure device or confirm that the device remains properly secured.
17. Ventilate patient at proper rate and volume while observing capnography/capnometry and pulse oximeter.

Emergency Surgical Airway

1. Assemble and test all the necessary equipment.
2. Take appropriate body substance isolation precautions.
3. Assess the upper airway for visible obstruction.
4. Identify the cricothyroid membrane between the thyroid and cricoid cartilages.
5. Identify the site of the skin incision.
6. Palpate the cricothyroid membrane and (while stabilizing the cartilage) make a vertical incision through skin directly over the cricothyroid membrane.
7. While continuing to stabilize the larynx, use the scalpel or a hemostat to cut or poke through the cricothyroid membrane.
8. Insert the tips of the hemostat through the opening and open the jaws to dilate the opening. A tracheal hook may also be used for this purpose, but care should be exercised as these hooks place the ET/trach balloon at risk.
9. Insert the ET tube between the jaws of the hemostat; the tube should be in the trachea and directed toward the lungs.
10. Inflate the cuff.
11. Check for air exchange and verify placement of the tube by listening and feeling for air passing in and out of the tube, causing the tube to mist, and looking for bilateral rise and fall of the chest.
12. If the position is correct, secure the tube with tape or a commercial tube-securing device.
13. Apply a dressing to further protect the tube and incision site.
14. Monitor the casualty's respirations. Ventilate if required.

REFERENCES AND RESOURCES

Collopy KT. Surgical cricothyrotomies in prehospital care. *EMS World*. 2015; January. https://www.emsworld.com/magazine/ems/issue/2015/jan. Accessed February 7, 2019.

Frerk C, Mitchell VS, McNarry AF, Mendonca C, Bhagrath R, Patel A, O'Sullivan EP, Woodall NM, Ahmad I, Difficult Airway Society intubation guidelines working group. Difficult Airway Society 2015 guidelines for management of unanticipated difficult intubation in adults. *Br J Anaesth*. 2015;115(6): 827-848.

Jagannathan N, Ramsey MA, White MC, Sohn L. An update on newer pediatric supraglottic airways with recommendations for clinical use. *Paediatrc Anaesth*. 2015;25(4):334-345.

National Association of Emergency Medical Technicians. *PHTLS: Prehospital Trauma Life Support*. 9th ed. Burlington, MA: Public Safety Group; 2019.

Otten EJ, Montgomery HR, Butler FK Jr. Extraglottic airways in tactical combat casualty care: TCCC guidelines change 17-01 28 August 2017. *J Spec Oper Med*. 2017;17(4):19-28.

Ryan JM, Hopperus Buma APCC, Beadling CW, Mozumder A, Nott DM, Rich NM, Henny W, MacGarty D (Eds.). *Conflict and Catastrophe Medicine: A Practical Guide*. 3rd ed. Switzerland: Springer Nature: 2014.

United Nations Department of Safety and Security. UN Security Officers' Emergency Trauma Bag/Basic First Aid (ETB/BFA). http://unesco.org.pk/documents/Basic%20Field%20Trauma%20Procedures.pdf. Accessed February 7, 2019.

LESSON 5

Indirect Threat Care/Warm Zone: Respiration/Breathing

LESSON OBJECTIVES

- Discuss the use of chest seals.
- Discuss the signs and symptoms of a tension pneumothorax.
- Discuss evidence-based changes in anatomic sites for needle decompression.
- Discuss indications for bilateral needle decompression for casualties in cardiac arrest.
- Discuss special considerations for needle decompression for pediatric casualties.

Overview of Respiration/Breathing in Indirect Threat Care/Warm Zone

After the tactical emergency casualty care (TECC) provider establishes and maintains an effective airway, the next clinical step is to assure adequate ventilation. The level of intervention will be based on the patient's clinical condition and the tactical situation within the indirect threat care/warm zone. Remember that the tactical situation could suddenly deteriorate into a direct threat/hot zone and require immediate movement of patient and caregiver.

Anatomy and Physiology of Breathing

The airway is a pathway that leads atmospheric air through the nose, mouth, pharynx, trachea, and bronchi to the alveoli. With each breath, the average 70-kg (150-lb) adult takes in approximately 500 milliliters (ml) of air. The airway system holds up to 150 ml of air that never actually reaches the alveoli to participate in the critical gas-exchange process. The space in which this air is held is known as dead space. The air inside this dead space is not available to the body to be used for oxygenation.

With each breath, air is drawn into the lungs. The movement of air into and out of the alveoli results from changes in intrathoracic pressure generated by the contraction and relaxation of specific muscle groups. The primary muscle of breathing is the diaphragm. Normally, the muscle fibers of the diaphragm shorten when a stimulus is received from the brain. In addition to the diaphragm, the external intercostal muscles help pull the ribs forward and upward. This flattening of the diaphragm along with the action of the intercostal muscles is an active movement that creates a negative pressure inside the thoracic cavity. This negative pressure causes atmospheric air to enter the intact pulmonary tree (**Figure 5-1**).

Other muscles attached to the chest wall can also contribute to the creation of this negative pressure; these include the sternocleidomastoid and scalene muscles. The use of these secondary muscles becomes evident as the work of breathing increases in the trauma patient. In contrast, exhalation is normally a passive process in nature, caused by the relaxation of the diaphragm and chest wall muscles and the elastic recoil of these structures. However, exhalation can become active as breathing becomes more difficult.

Generating this negative pressure during inspiration requires an intact chest wall. For example, in the trauma patient, a wound that creates an open pathway between the outside atmosphere and the thoracic cavity can result in air being pulled in through the open

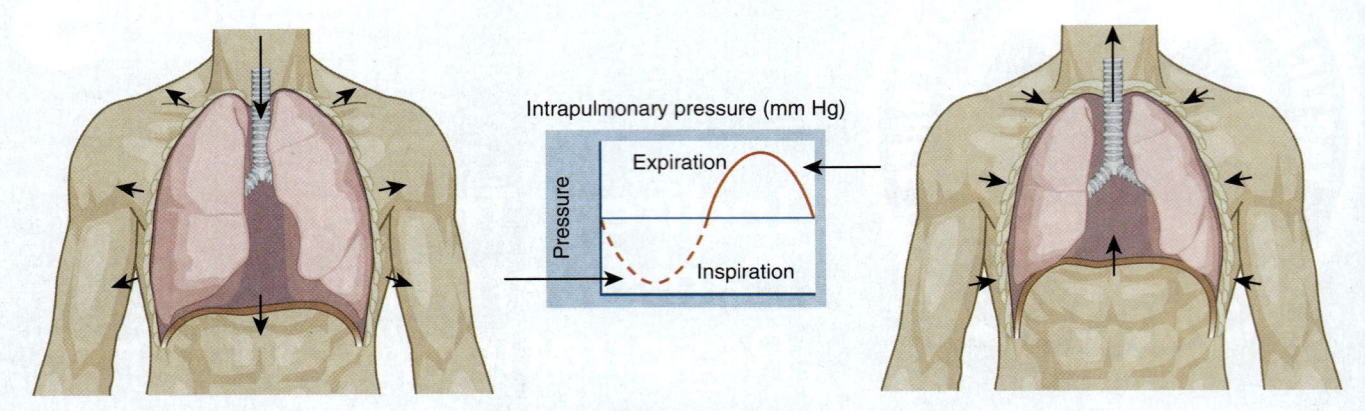

Figure 5-1 Graph showing the relationship of intrapulmonary pressure during the phases of ventilation.
© Jones & Bartlett Learning.

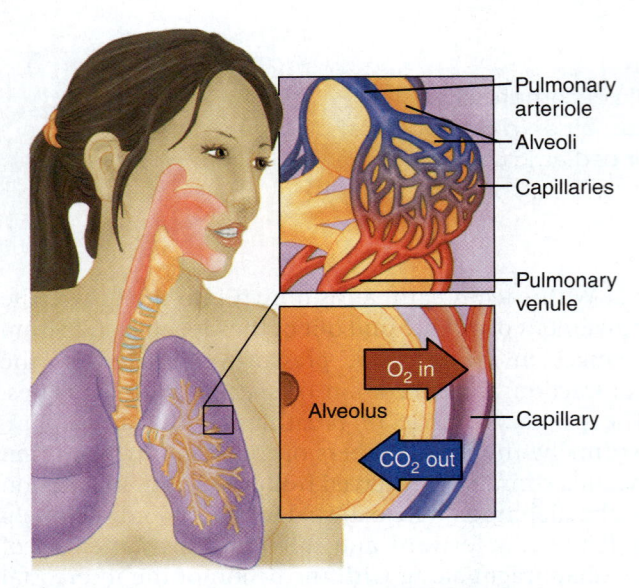

Figure 5-2 Diffusion of oxygen and carbon dioxide across the alveolar-capillary membrane of the alveoli in the lungs.
© Jones & Bartlett Learning.

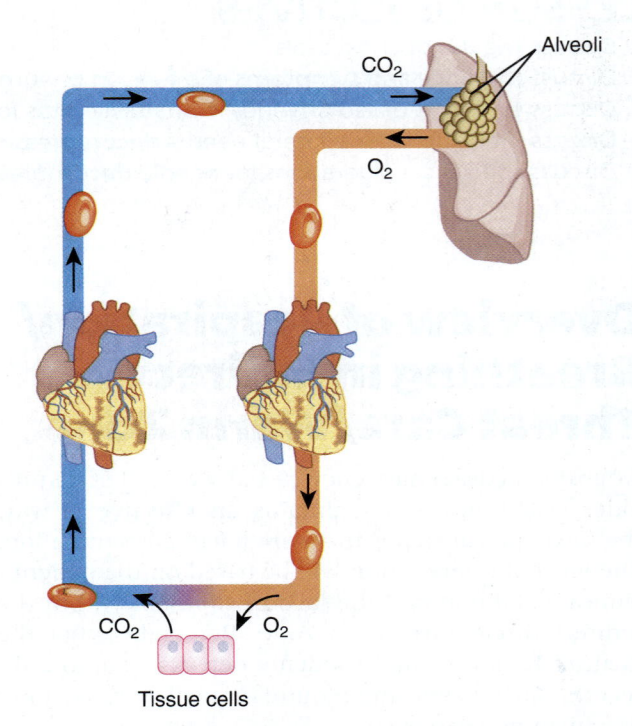

Figure 5-3 Oxygen (O_2) moves into the red blood cells from the alveoli. The O_2 is transferred to the tissue cell on the hemoglobin molecule. After leaving the hemoglobin molecule, the O_2 travels into the tissue cell. Carbon dioxide (CO_2) travels in the reverse direction, but not on the hemoglobin molecule. It travels in the plasma as CO_2.
© National Association of Emergency Medical Technicians (NAEMT).

wound rather than into the lungs. Damage to the bony structure of the chest wall may also compromise the patient's ability to generate the needed negative pressure required for adequate ventilation.

When atmospheric air reaches the alveoli, oxygen moves from the alveoli, across the alveolar-capillary membrane, and into the red blood cells (RBCs) (**Figure 5-2**).

The circulatory system then delivers the oxygen-carrying RBCs to the body tissues, where oxygen is used as fuel for metabolism. As oxygen is transferred from inside the alveoli across the cell wall and capillary endothelium, through the plasma, and into the RBCs, carbon dioxide is exchanged in the opposite direction, from the blood to the alveoli. Carbon dioxide, which is carried dissolved in the plasma (approximately 10%), bound to proteins (mostly hemoglobin in the RBCs [approximately 20%]), and as bicarbonate (approximately 70%), moves from the bloodstream, across the alveolar-capillary membrane, and into the alveoli, where it is eliminated during exhalation (**Figure 5-3**).

On completion of this exchange, the oxygenated RBCs and plasma with a low carbon dioxide level return to the left side of the heart to be pumped to all the cells in the body.

Once at the cell, the oxygenated RBCs deliver their oxygen, which the cells then use for aerobic metabolism. Carbon dioxide, a by-product of aerobic metabolism, is released into the blood plasma. Deoxygenated blood returns to the right side of the heart. The blood is pumped to the lungs, where it is again supplied with oxygen, and the carbon dioxide is eliminated by diffusion. The oxygen is transported mostly by hemoglobin in the RBCs themselves, whereas the carbon dioxide is transported in the three ways previously mentioned: in the plasma, bound to proteins such as hemoglobin, and buffered as bicarbonate.

The Oxygenation and Ventilation Process

The alveoli must be constantly replenished with a fresh supply of air that contains an adequate amount of oxygen. This replenishment of air, known as ventilation, is also essential for the elimination of carbon dioxide. The oxygenation process involves three phases:

1. **External respiration** is the transfer of oxygen molecules from air to the blood. Air contains oxygen (21%) and nitrogen (79%). All alveolar oxygen exists as free gas; therefore, each oxygen molecule exerts pressure. Increasing the percentage of oxygen in the inspired atmosphere will increase alveolar oxygen pressure or tension. When supplemental oxygen is provided, the ratio of oxygen in each inspiration increases, causing an increase in the amount of oxygen in each alveolus. This, in turn, will increase the amount of gas that gets transferred to blood because the amount of gas that will enter a liquid is directly related to the pressure it exerts. The greater the pressure of the gas, the greater the amount of that gas that will be absorbed into the fluid.
2. **Oxygen delivery** is the result of oxygen transfer from the atmosphere to the RBCs during ventilation and the transportation of these RBCs to the tissues via the cardiovascular system. The volume of oxygen consumed by the body in 1 minute in order to maintain energy production is known as oxygen consumption and depends on adequate cardiac output and the delivery of oxygen to the cells by RBCs. The RBCs could be described as the body's "oxygen tankers." These oxygen tankers move along the vascular system "highways" to "off-load" their oxygen supply at the body's distribution points, the capillary beds.
3. **Internal (cellular) respiration** is the movement, or diffusion, of oxygen from the RBCs into the tissue cells. Metabolism normally occurs through glycolysis and the Krebs cycle to produce energy. While understanding the specific details of these processes is not necessary, it is important to have a general understanding of their role in energy production. Because the actual exchange of oxygen between the RBCs and the tissues occurs in the thin-walled capillaries, any factor that interrupts a supply of oxygen will disrupt this cycle. A major factor in this regard is the amount of fluid (or edema) located between the alveolar walls, the capillary walls, and the wall of the tissue cells (also known as the interstitial space). Overhydration of the vascular space with crystalloid, which leaks out of the vascular system into the interstitial space within 30 to 45 minutes after administration, is a major problem during resuscitation. Supplemental oxygen can help overcome some of these factors. The tissues and cells cannot consume adequate amounts of oxygen if adequate amounts are not available.

Pathophysiology

Trauma can affect the respiratory system's ability to adequately provide oxygen and eliminate carbon dioxide in the following ways:

- Hypoxemia (decreased oxygen level in the blood) can result from decreased diffusion of oxygen across the alveolar-capillary membrane.
- Hypoxia (deficient tissue oxygenation) can be caused by:
  - The inability of the air to reach the capillaries, usually because the airway is obstructed or the alveoli are filled with fluid or debris
  - Decreased blood flow to the alveoli
  - Decreased blood flow to the tissue cells
- Hypoventilation can result from:
  - Obstruction of airflow through the upper and lower airways
  - Decreased expansion of the lungs as a result of direct injury to the chest wall or lungs
  - Loss of ventilatory drive, usually because of decreased neurologic function, most often after a traumatic brain injury

Hyperventilation can cause vasoconstriction, which can be especially detrimental in the management of the traumatic brain-injured patient.

Hypoventilation results from the reduction of minute volume. If left untreated, hypoventilation results in carbon dioxide buildup, acidosis, and eventually death. Management involves improving the patient's ventilatory rate and depth by correcting existing airway problems and assisting ventilation as appropriate.

> **CHECK YOUR KNOWLEDGE**
>
> **Generating negative pressure during inspiration requires a(n):**
>
> a. intact chest wall.
> b. adequate cardiac output.
> c. systolic blood pressure above 50 mm Hg.
> d. intact alveoli structure.

Open Pneumothorax

In penetrating injuries of the chest, objects of varying size and type traverse the chest wall, enter the thoracic cavity, and possibly injure the organs within the thorax. Normally, no space exists between the pleural membranes. However, when a penetrating wound creates a communication between the chest cavity and the outside world, air can enter the pleural space through the wound during inspiration when the pressure inside the chest is lower than the pressure outside the chest. Air may be further encouraged to enter a wound if the resistance to airflow through the wound is less than that through the airways. Air in the pleural space (pneumothorax) disrupts the adherence between the pleural membranes created by the thin film of pleural fluid. Together, these processes cause the lung to collapse, preventing effective ventilation within the collapsed portion. Penetrating wounds result in an open pneumothorax only when the size of the chest wall defect is large enough that the surrounding tissues do not close the wound at least partially during inspiration and/or expiration (**Figure 5-4**).

Wounds of the lung caused by a penetrating object allow air to escape from the lung into the pleural space and result in collapse of the lung. In either case, the patient becomes short of breath. To make up for the lost ventilation capacity, the respiratory center will stimulate more rapid breathing. This increases the work of breathing. The patient may be able to tolerate the increased workload for a time, but if not recognized and treated, the patient is at risk for ventilatory failure, which will be manifested by increasing respiratory distress as the carbon dioxide levels in the blood rise and the oxygen levels fall.

An open pneumothorax involves air entering the pleural space, causing the lung to collapse. A defect in the chest wall that results in a communication between the outside air and the pleural space is the hallmark of an open pneumothorax. Injuries leading to open pneumothorax include gunshot wounds, shotgun blasts, stabbings, impalements, and, rarely, blunt trauma. When the patient attempts to inhale, air crosses the open wound and enters the pleural space because of the negative pressure created in the thoracic cavity as the muscles of respiration contract. In larger wounds, there may be free flow of air in and out of the pleural space with the different phases of respiration. Audible noise is often created as air travels in and out of the hole in the chest wall; thus, this type of wound has been referred to as a "sucking chest wound" (**Figure 5-5**).

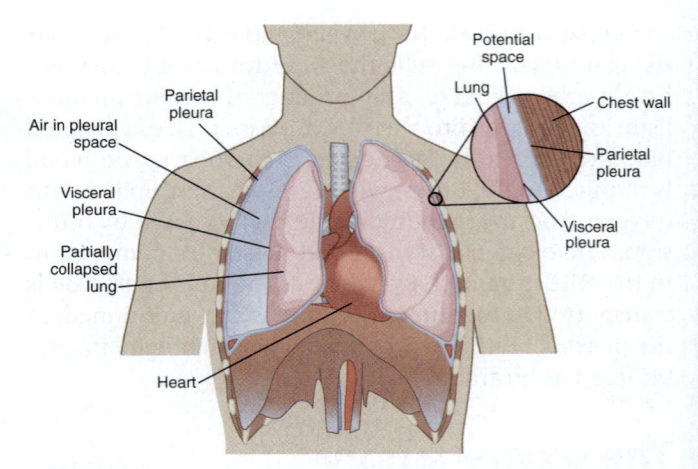

Figure 5-4 Air in the pleural space forces the lung in, decreasing the amount that can be ventilated and, therefore, decreasing oxygenation of the blood leaving the lung.
© National Association of Emergency Medical Technicians (NAEMT).

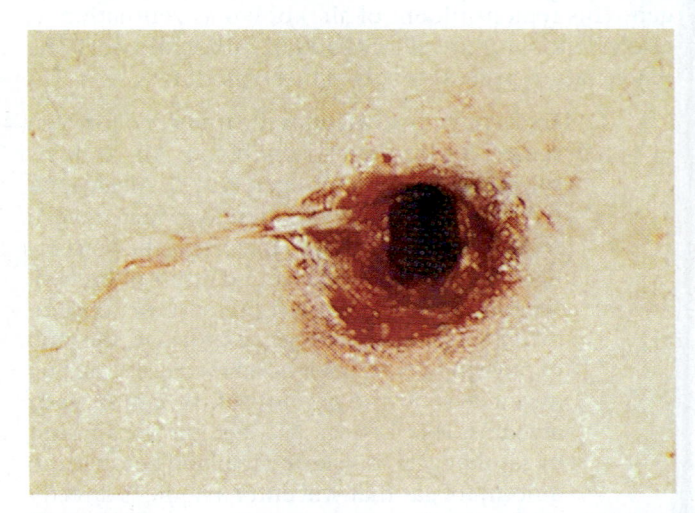

Figure 5-5 A gunshot or stab wound to the chest produces a hole in the chest wall through which air can flow both into and out of the pleural cavity.
Courtesy of Norman McSwain, MD, FACS, NREMT-P.

Assessment and Management of an Open Pneumothorax

Assessment of the patient with an open pneumothorax generally reveals obvious respiratory distress. The patient is typically anxious and tachypneic (breathing rapidly). The pulse rate is elevated and potentially

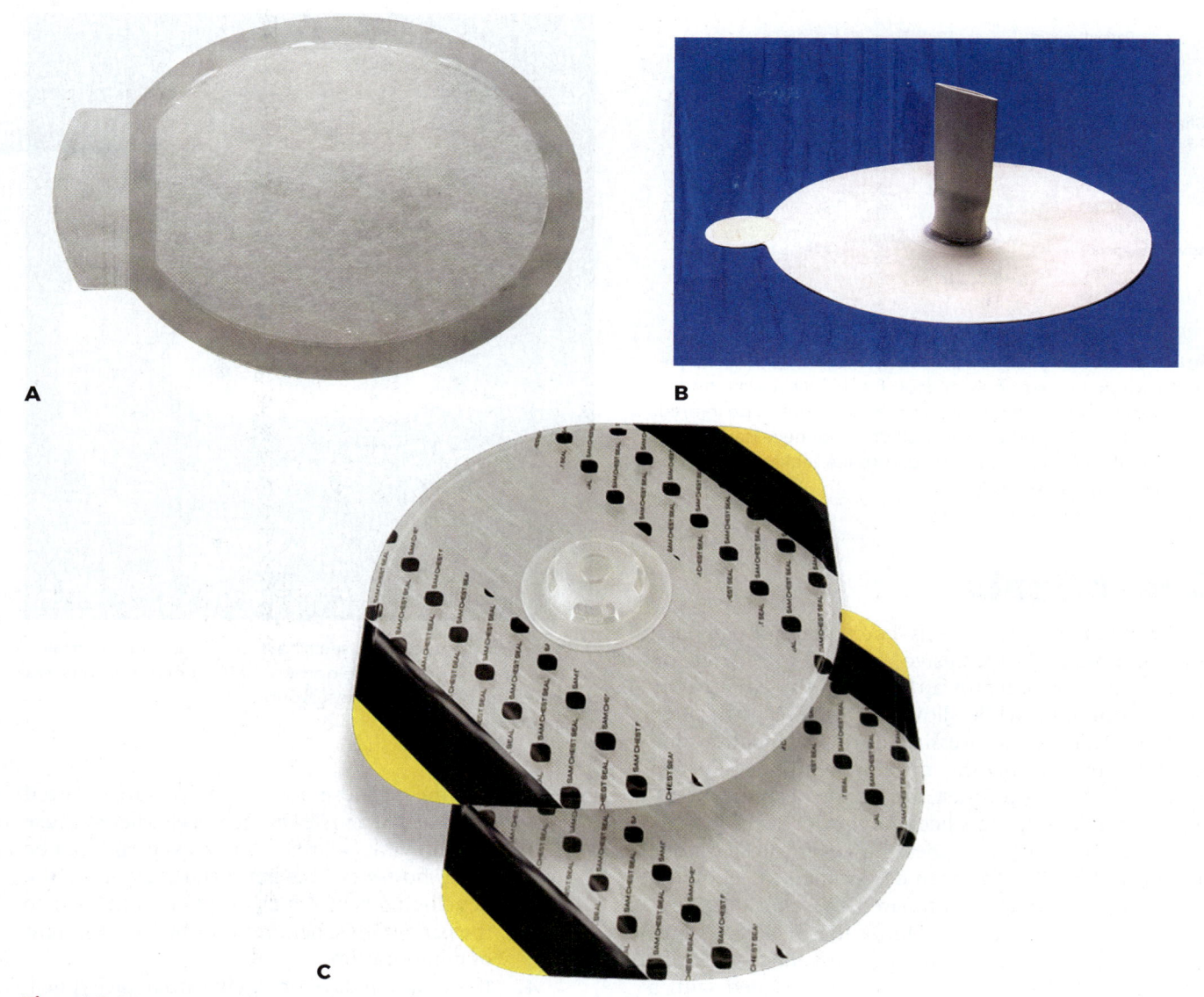

Figure 5-6 **A.** Halo chest seal. **B.** Asherman chest seal. **C.** SAM chest seal.

A: Reproduced with permission from Halo Chest Seal. Retrieved from https://www.halochestseal.com/; B: Image courtesy of Teleflex Incorporated. © (2019) Teleflex Incorporated. All rights reserved; C: Reproduced with permission from SAM Chest Seal, SAM Medical. Retrieved from https://www.sammedical.com/products/sam-chest-seal

thready. Examination of the chest wall reveals the wound, which may make audible sucking sounds during inspiration, with bubbling during expiration.

Initial management of an open pneumothorax involves sealing the defect in the chest wall and administering supplemental oxygen. Airflow through the wound into the pleural cavity is prevented by applying an occlusive dressing using commercial products such as the Halo, Asherman, or SAM chest seals or improvised methods such as application of aluminum foil or plastic wrap; unlike plain gauze, these materials do not allow airflow through them (**Figure 5-6**)

A patient with an open pneumothorax virtually always has an injury to the underlying lung, allowing for two sources of air leak, the first being the hole in the chest wall and the second being the hole in the lung. Even if an injury to the chest wall is sealed with an occlusive dressing, air leakage into the pleural space can continue from the injured lung, setting the stage for the development of a tension pneumothorax (**Figure 5-7**).

> **CHECK YOUR KNOWLEDGE**
>
> **A casualty with an open pneumothorax always:**
> a. requires spinal immobilization.
> b. presents with distended neck veins.
> c. requires evaluation for cardiac tamponade.
> d. has an injury to the underlying lung.

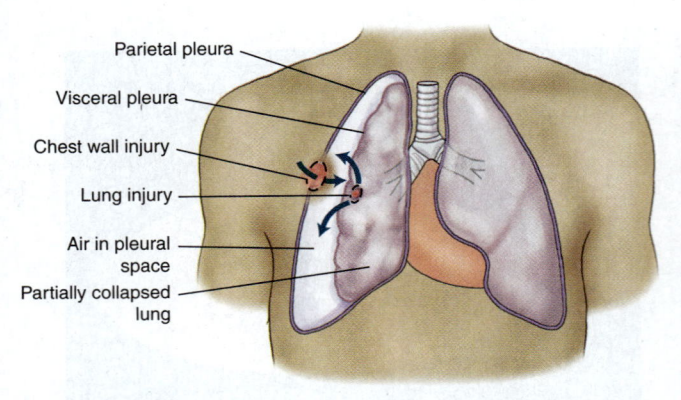

Figure 5-7 Because of the proximity of the chest wall to the lung, it would be extremely difficult for the chest wall to be injured by penetrating trauma and the lung not to be injured. Stopping the hole in the chest wall does not necessarily decrease air leakage into the pleural space; leakage can come from the lung just as easily.
© National Association of Emergency Medical Technicians (NAEMT).

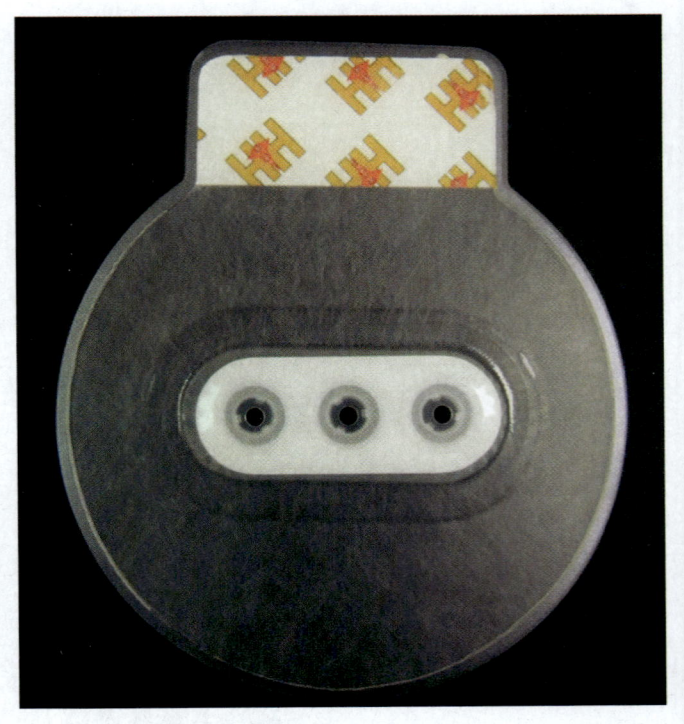

Figure 5-8 Vented chest seals have been shown in animal studies to prevent the development of tension pneumothorax after sealing of an open chest wound.
Courtesy of H & H Medical Corporation.

Chest Seals

The traditional teaching has been that for an open pneumothorax, the occlusive dressing is secured on three sides. This prevents airflow into the chest cavity during inspiration while allowing air to escape through the loose side of the dressing during exhalation and hopefully preventing the development of a tension pneumothorax. In contrast, taping the occlusive dressing on all four sides has been advocated as preferable to taping only on three sides; however, no definitive answer to this issue has been determined.

A study in animals compared the physiologic response of an open pneumothorax that has been completely sealed with a commercial unvented occlusive dressing to the response in those cases sealed with a vented dressing. This study showed that both seals improved the respiratory physiology associated with an open pneumothorax; however, the vented seal prevented the development of tension pneumothorax, which the unvented seal did not. This finding has led the military's Committee on Tactical Combat Casualty Care to recommend that, if available, a vented chest seal is preferred over an unvented chest seal (**Figure 5-8**). An unvented chest seal is an acceptable alternative if the vented type is not available; however, the patient must be carefully observed for the subsequent development of a tension pneumothorax.

In view of this research, Prehospital Trauma Life Support (PHTLS) now recommends the following approach to the management of an open pneumothorax:

1. Place a vented chest seal over the open chest wound.
2. If a vented seal is not available, place a plastic or foil square over the wound and tape on three sides.
3. If none of these are available, an unvented chest seal or a material such as petroleum gauze that prevents ingress and egress of air may be used; however, this approach may allow the development of a tension pneumothorax, so the patient must be carefully observed for signs of deterioration.
4. If the patient develops tachycardia, tachypnea, or other indications of respiratory distress, remove the dressing for a few seconds and assist ventilations as necessary.
5. If respiratory distress continues, assume the development of a tension pneumothorax and attempt to "burp" the seal/dressing. However, this may not be effective due to a variety of factors. If "burp" is unsuccessful, perform a needle thoracostomy on the injured side using a large-bore (10-14 gauge needle) that is a minimum 3.25" in length in the fifth intercostal space along the anterior axillary line or in the second intercostal space at the midclavicular line.

If possible, allow the casualty to seek a position of comfort, such as sitting upright. If the casualty wants to lie down, lay the casualty with the injured side down to reduce the respiratory effort from the collapsed lung.

If these measures fail to support the patient adequately, endotracheal intubation and positive-pressure ventilation may be necessary, if the tactical situation allows. If positive pressure is utilized and a dressing has been applied to seal the open wound, the TECC provider needs to monitor the patient carefully for the development of a tension pneumothorax. If signs of increasing respiratory distress develop, the dressing over the wound should be removed to allow for decompression of any accumulating tension. If this is ineffective, needle decompression and positive-pressure ventilation should be considered, if not already employed.

In those situations where positive-pressure ventilation is being performed, the wound does not need to be sealed. The positive-pressure ventilation effectively manages the pathophysiology usually associated with the open pneumothorax by ventilating the lung directly.

Tension Pneumothorax

Tension pneumothorax is a life-threatening emergency. As air continues to enter the pleural space without any exit or release, intrathoracic pressure builds up. As intrathoracic pressure rises, ventilatory compromise increases and venous return to the heart decreases. The decreasing cardiac output coupled with worsening gas exchange results in profound shock. The increasing pressure on the injured side of the chest may eventually push the structures in the mediastinum toward the other side of the chest (**Figure 5-9**).

This distortion of anatomy may further impede venous return to the heart through the kinking of the inferior vena cava as it passes through the diaphragm. Additionally, inflation of the lung on the uninjured side is increasingly restricted, and further respiratory compromise results.

Any patient with thoracic injury is at risk for development of a tension pneumothorax. Patients at particular risk are those who likely have a pneumothorax (e.g., patient with signs of rib fracture), those who have a known pneumothorax (e.g., patient with a penetrating wound to the chest), and those with chest injury who are undergoing positive-pressure ventilation. These patients must be continuously monitored for signs of increasing respiratory distress associated with circulatory impairment and rapidly transported to an appropriate facility.

Assessment and Management of a Tension Pneumothorax

The findings during assessment depend on how much pressure has accumulated in the pleural space. Initially, patients will exhibit apprehension and discomfort. They will generally complain of chest pain and difficulty breathing. As the tension pneumothorax worsens, they will exhibit increasing agitation, tachypnea, and respiratory distress. In severe cases, cyanosis and apnea may occur.

The priority in management involves decompressing the tension pneumothorax. Decompression should be performed when the following three findings are present:

1. Worsening respiratory distress or difficulty ventilating with a bag-mask device
2. Unilateral decreased or absent breath sounds
3. Decompensated shock (systolic blood pressure <90 mm Hg with a narrowed pulse pressure)

Depending upon the clinical setting and the training level of the prehospital care provider, several options for pleural decompression exist. If decompression is not an option (i.e., only basic life support [BLS] available and no occlusive dressing to remove), rapid transport to an appropriate facility while administering high-concentration oxygen (fraction of inspired oxygen [Fio$_2$] >85%) is imperative. Positive-pressure ventilatory assistance should be used only if the patient is hypoxic and fails to respond to supplemental oxygen, as this situation may rapidly worsen the tension pneumothorax. Assisting ventilations may result in air accumulating more rapidly in the pleural space. If advanced life support (ALS) intercept is an option, it should be accomplished if the intercept will be faster than delivery to an appropriate facility.

In the patient with an open pneumothorax, if an occluding dressing has been applied, it should be

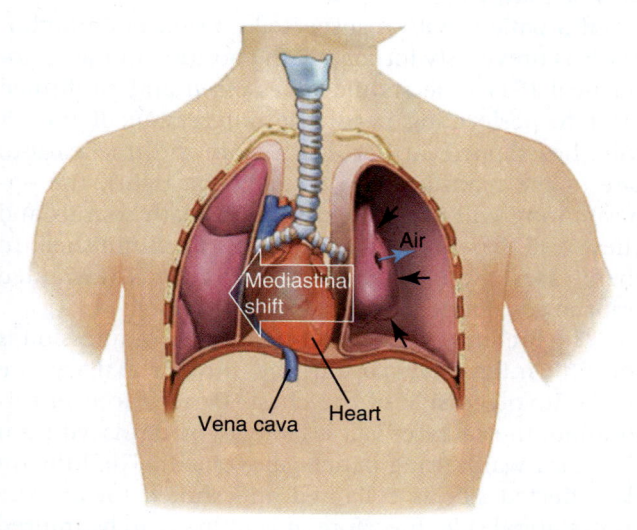

Figure 5-9 Tension pneumothorax. If the amount of air trapped in the pleural space continues to increase, not only will the lung on the affected side collapse, but the mediastinum will shift to the opposite side. The lung on the opposite side is then compressed and intrathoracic pressure increases, which kinks the vena cava and decreases blood return to the heart.

© National Association of Emergency Medical Technicians (NAEMT).

briefly opened or removed. This should allow the tension pneumothorax to decompress through the wound with a rush of air. This procedure may need to be repeated periodically during transport if symptoms of tension pneumothorax recur. If removing the dressing for several seconds is ineffective or if there is no open wound, an ALS provider may proceed with a needle thoracostomy.

> **CHECK YOUR KNOWLEDGE**
>
> **Which is a late sign with tension pneumothorax?**
>
> a. anxiety
> b. diminished/absent breath sounds
> c. tracheal deviation
> d. unequal chest rise and fall

Needle Decompression

Insertion of a needle into the pleural space of the affected side permits accumulated air, under pressure, to escape. While studies in human patients have primarily been anecdotal, needle decompression has been shown to be effective in an animal model. The immediate improvement in oxygenation and in ease of ventilation may be lifesaving.

If a patient with a suspected tension pneumothorax was previously intubated, the position of the endotracheal (ET) tube should be assessed and confirmed prior to performing needle decompression. If the ET tube has slipped farther down from the trachea into one of the main bronchi (usually the right), the opposite lung will not be ventilated. Breath sounds and chest wall expansion may be markedly diminished. In these cases, repositioning of the ET tube is warranted prior to considering needle decompression.

The preferred location for needle decompression is the fifth intercostal space at the anterior axillary line of the involved side of the chest. Once placed in this location, the catheter is less likely to be displaced from the chest wall during patient movement. The lung on the affected side is collapsed and shifted toward the contralateral side; therefore, it is unlikely to be injured during the procedure. The needle and catheter should be advanced until the return of a rush of air is achieved and advanced no farther. Once the decompression is achieved, the catheter is taped to the chest to prevent dislodgement. Improper placement (location or depth) may result in injuries to the lungs, heart, or great vessels (**Figure 5-10**).

BOX 5-1

Signs of Tension Pneumothorax

Although the following signs are frequently discussed with a tension pneumothorax, many may not be present or are difficult to identify in the field.

Observation

- *Cyanosis* may be difficult to see in the field. Poor lighting, variation in skin color, and dirt and blood associated with trauma often render this sign unreliable.
- *Distended neck veins* are described as a classic sign of tension pneumothorax. However, because a patient with a tension pneumothorax may also have lost a considerable amount of blood, distended neck veins may not be prominent.

Palpation

- *Subcutaneous emphysema* is a common finding. As the pressure builds up within the chest cavity, air will begin to dissect through the tissues of the chest wall. Because tension pneumothorax involves significantly elevated intrathoracic pressure, subcutaneous emphysema can often be palpated across the entire chest wall and neck and sometimes can involve the abdominal wall and face as well.
- *Tracheal deviation* is usually a late sign. Even when it is present, it can be difficult to diagnose by physical examination. In the neck, the trachea is bound to the cervical spine by fascial and other supporting structures; thus, the deviation of the trachea is more of an intrathoracic phenomenon, although deviation may be palpated in the jugular notch if it is severe. Tracheal deviation is not often noted in the prehospital environment.

Auscultation

- *Decreased breath sounds on the injured side*. The most helpful part of the physical examination is checking for decreased breath sounds on the side of the injury. However, to use this sign, the prehospital care provider must be able to distinguish between normal and decreased sounds. Such differentiation requires a great deal of practice. Listening to breath sounds during every patient contact will help.

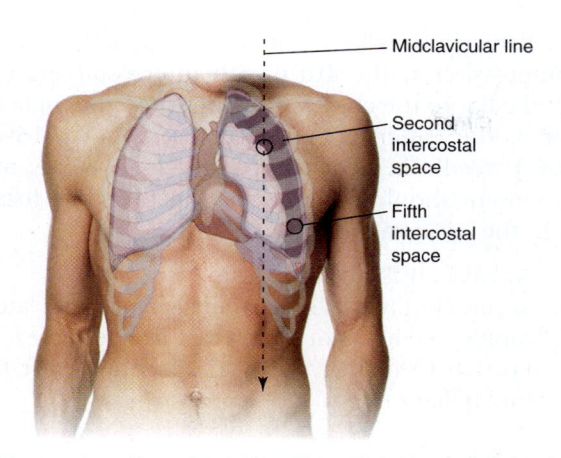

Figure 5-10 Needle decompression of the thoracic cavity is most easily accomplished and produces the least chance for complication if it is done at the anterior axillary line through the fifth intercostal space.
© MariyaL/Shutterstock.

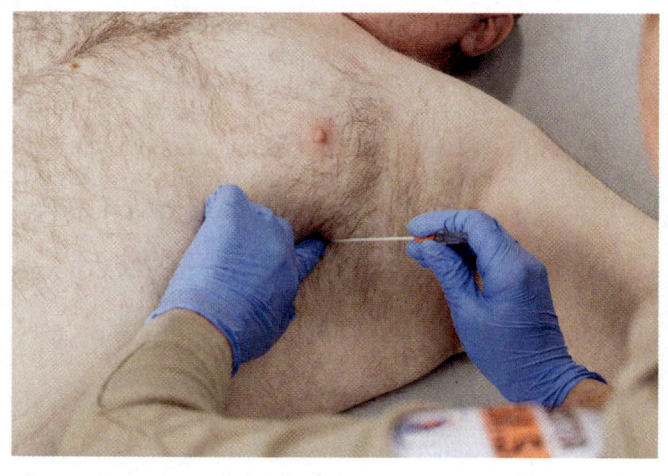

Figure 5-11 Needle decompression.
© Jones & Bartlett Learning. Photographed by Darren Stahlman.

Several studies questioned the previously preferred location for placement of the second or third intercostal space at the midclavicular line, noting that chest wall thickness in the midclavicular line is often greater than the length of the catheter commonly used for decompression. Evidence suggests that placement of the catheter in the fifth intercostal space at the anterior axillary line could provide greater success. A study using computed tomography (CT) scan to review chest wall thickness of trauma patients noted an average chest wall thickness in the midclavicular line to be 46 mm (right) and 45 mm (left). In the same patients, the average chest wall thickness was 33 mm (right) and 32 mm (left) in the anterior axillary line. The study's authors noted that needle decompression using a standard 5-cm needle would fail in 42.5% of cases in the midclavicular line versus only 16.7% in the anterior axillary line. The authors also noted in a cadaveric study that needle decompression in the fifth intercostal space, midaxillary line resulted in 100% successful placement into the thoracic cavity compared to only 57.5% in the midclavicular line.

Decompression in the midclavicular line has the advantage of ease of access for the prehospital care provider. However, there is a higher risk of inadequately decompressing the chest or failing entirely due to inadequate catheter length or suboptimal position with the lateral approach. As noted earlier, chest wall thickness often results in the catheter never actually entering the thoracic cavity. Advantages of the anterior axillary placement of the catheter include its relative safety and efficacy.

Regardless of the method chosen, decompression should be performed with a large-bore (10-14 gauge) Intravenous (IV) needle that is at least 3.25" in length.

Careful monitoring of the patient following the procedure is mandatory. A recent review noted a 26% mechanical failure rate due to kinking, obstruction, or dislodgement, with 43% of attempts ultimately failing to relieve the tension pneumothorax (**Figure 5-11**).

TECC Needle Decompression Procedure

1. Prepare equipment.
2. Take body substance isolation precautions.
3. Identify the fifth intercostal space on the chest wall at the anterior axillary line on the same side as the injury.
4. The needle to be used for the procedure is a 3.25-inch, 14-gauge needle.
5. Clean the site with an antimicrobial solution (alcohol or Betadine).
6. Insert the needle into the chest.
   a. Remove the plastic cap from the 3.25-inch, 14-gauge needle. Also remove the cover to the needle's flash chamber.
   b. For lateral decompression: Insert the needle in the fifth intercostal space perpendicular to the chest wall, at approximately the anterior axillary line.
   c. Ensure that the needle entry into the chest is lateral to the nipple line and is not directed toward the heart.
   d. For anterior decompression: Insert the needle into the skin over the superior border of the third rib, midclavicular line, and direct the needle into the second intercostal space at a 90-degree angle.
   e. As the needle enters the pleural space, a "pop" is felt, followed by a possible hiss of

air. Ensure that the needle is advanced all the way to the hub.
  f. Remove the needle, leaving the catheter in place.
  g. If the tension pneumothorax reoccurs (as noted by return of respiratory distress), repeat the needle decompression on the injured side.
7. Stabilize the catheter hub to the chest wall with ½-inch gauze tape.
8. Listen for increased breath sounds or observe decreased respiratory distress.
9. Remove gloves and dispose of them appropriately.

Assessing the Effectiveness of Needle Decompression

This procedure, when successfully performed, converts the tension pneumothorax into a negligible open pneumothorax. The relief to respiratory effort far outweighs the negative effect of the open pneumothorax. Because the diameter of the decompression catheter is significantly smaller than the patient's airway, it is unlikely that any air movement through the catheter will significantly compromise ventilatory effort. Continued provision of supplemental oxygen, as well as ventilatory support as needed, is appropriate. Proper documentation of the indications for needle decompression is important, as the casualty may require a subsequent chest tube or further interventions.

Bilateral Needle Decompression for Traumatic Cardiac Arrest

In situations in which a patient with torso trauma presents with no pulse or respirations, the Committee for Tactical Emergency Casualty Care recommends bilateral needle decompression to rule out tension pneumothorax as the cause of respiratory and cardiac arrest.

Pediatric Tension Pneumothorax

Signs and symptoms of pediatric tension pneumothorax are the same as those for an adult—progressive distress with known or suspected torso trauma.

As with an adult casualty, a pediatric patient with a tension pneumothorax typically presents in shock with severe respiratory distress and may or may not have tracheal deviation to the unaffected side. If the pneumothorax is due to trauma, look for contusions or abrasions on the chest wall or a small puncture wound that does not allow free movement of air between the outside and the pleural cavity.

Pediatric needle decompression uses the lateral decompression at the 4th or 5th intercostal space, perpendicular to the chest wall, anterior to the midaxillary line as the preferred approach. Use a 14- to 16-gauge (1.5") needle in pediatric patients <13 years of age. Treatment should be performed in the same locations as in the adult casualty:

- Always on the injured side
- Second intercostal space midclavicular line lateral to nipple line and not directed at the heart
- Fourth to fifth intercostal space anterior to the midaxillary line

> **CHECK YOUR KNOWLEDGE**
>
> **A needle/catheter size appropriate for decompression is _____ gauge**
>
> a. 8
> b. 14
> c. 18
> d. 22

Summary

- Treat open pneumothoraces with vented chest seals.
- Tension pneumothorax is one of the leading causes of preventable death in the tactical setting.
- Treatment entails letting the trapped air escape.
- Anticipation and recognition are vital.
- Remember the dynamic nature of active shooter/hostile event (ASHE) situations!

Skill Station
Needle Decompression

1. Prepare equipment.
2. Take appropriate body substance isolation precautions.
3. Identify that the progressive respiratory distress is due to chest trauma.
4. Identify the fifth intercostal space on the chest wall at the anterior axillary line on the same side as the injury.
5. Identify that the needle to be used for the procedure is a 3.25-inch, 14-gauge needle.
6. Identify the importance of ensuring that the needle entry site is not medial to the nipple line.
7. Clean the site with an antimicrobial solution (alcohol or Betadine).
8. Insert the needle into the chest.

a. Remove the plastic cap from the 3.25-inch, 14-gauge needle. Also remove the cover to the needle's flash chamber.
b. For lateral decompression: Insert the needle in the fifth intercostal space perpendicular to the chest wall, anterior to the midaxillary line.
c. For anterior decompression: Insert the needle into the skin over the superior border of the third rib, at the midclavicular line, and direct the needle into the second intercostal space at a 90-degree angle.
  i. Ensure that the needle entry into the chest is lateral to the nipple line and is not directed toward the heart.
d. As the needle enters the pleural space, ensure a "pop" is felt, followed by a possible hiss of air. Ensure that the needle is advanced all the way to the hub.
e. Remove the needle, leaving the catheter in place.
f. If the tension pneumothorax reoccurs (as noted by return of respiratory distress), repeat the needle decompression on the injured side.
9. Stabilize the catheter hub to the chest wall with a ½-inch gauze tape.
10. Listen for increased breath sounds or observe decreased respiratory distress.
11. Remove gloves and dispose of them appropriately.

REFERENCES AND RESOURCES

Ferrie EP, Collum N, McGovern S. The right place in the right space? Awareness of site for needle thoracocentesis. *Emerg Med J*. 2005;22:788-789.

Inaba K, Branco BC, Eckstein M, et al. Optimal positioning for emergent needle thoracostomy: a cadaver-based study. *J Trauma*. 2011;71:1099-1103.

Inaba K, Ives C, McClure K, et al. Radiologic evaluation of alternative sites for needle decompression of tension pneumothorax. *JAMA Surgery*. 2012;147(9): 813-818. doi:10.1001/archsurg.2012.751.

Kheirabadi BS, Terrazas IB, Koller A, Allen PB, Klemcke HG, Convertino VA, Dubick MA, Gerhardt RT, Blackbourne LH. Vented versus unvented chest seals for treatment of pneumothorax and prevention of tension pneumothorax in a swine model. *J Trauma Acute Care Surg*. 2013;75(1):150-156.

Kolinsky DC, Moy HP. Evidence-based EMS: needle decompression. Recent data may cause us to reconsider our preferred thoracostomy location. *EMS World*. 2015 Mar;44(3):28-30, 32-34.

Martin M, Satterly S, Inaba K, Blair K. Does needle thoracostomy provide adequate and effective decompression of tension pneumothorax? *J Trauma Acute Care Surg*. 2012;73(6):1412-1417.

National Association of Emergency Medical Technicians. *PHTLS: Prehospital Trauma Life Support*. 9th ed. Burlington, MA: Public Safety Group; 2019.

LESSON 6

Indirect Threat Care/Warm Zone: MARCH—Circulation

LESSON OBJECTIVES
- Discuss application of tourniquets during indirect threat care/warm zone.
- Discuss safe and effective hemorrhage control for partial and complete amputations.
- Discuss application of pelvic binders.
- Describe basic shock assessment and treatment.
- Discuss safe and effective venous access.
- Describe the use of tranexamic acid (TXA) in casualty care.
- Discuss the rationale and concepts of damage control resuscitation.
- Discuss the potential complications associated with resuscitation with normal saline.

Overview of Circulation in Indirect Threat Care

Once the airway and breathing are assured, the tactical emergency casualty care (TECC) provider reassesses the bleeding control initially applied while the casualty was in the direct threat/hot zone either by a caregiver or the casualty. Remember that the tactical situation could suddenly deteriorate, changing the indirect threat care/warm zone into a direct threat care/hot zone and requiring immediate movement of the patient and caregiver.

Tourniquet Assessment and Application in Indirect Threat Care/Warm Zone

Tourniquets work properly when compression of limb tissue stops arterial blood flow and no distal pulse is present. Well-designed tourniquets should be both easy to use and durable. Importantly, they should be mechanically effective enough to ensure occlusion of arterial blood flow without excessive pressure.

Tourniquet use is associated with characteristic complications. For instance, insufficient compression will stop only venous flow, trapping blood in the limb with potentially detrimental consequences. The trapped blood causes limb edema and loss of blood to the general circulation, which can potentially contribute to the onset of shock. Bleeding may actually increase with the development of venous hypertension. Other complications include ischemia, compression, and reperfusion injury. Muscle cells, in particular, may be more susceptible to ischemia and reperfusion effects after prolonged tourniquet use. Nerve compression may result in neuropathy and weakness; however, evidence suggests this nerve damage is typically minor and reversible.

The U.S. military, through the Tactical Combat Casualty Care (TCCC) program, recommends three tourniquets: the Combat Application Tourniquet (CAT), the Special Operations Forces Tactical Tourniquet (SOFTT), and the Emergency and Military Tourniquet. Testing by the military found that these three tourniquets were 100% effective in stopping arterial blood flow in the limbs of volunteers who applied their own tourniquets. The CAT and SOFTT use a strap and a windlass for tightening, and the Emergency and Military Tourniquet is a pneumatic tourniquet with an air bladder and an inflation bulb to produce compression. These three tourniquets are intended for use on thighs or upper arms (**Figure 6-1**).

A separate category of tourniquets, called junctional tourniquets, comprises devices designed to stop bleeding in the areas between the trunk and the limbs where

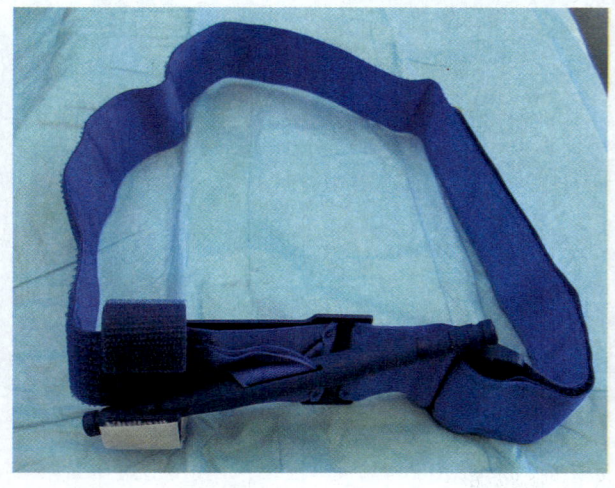

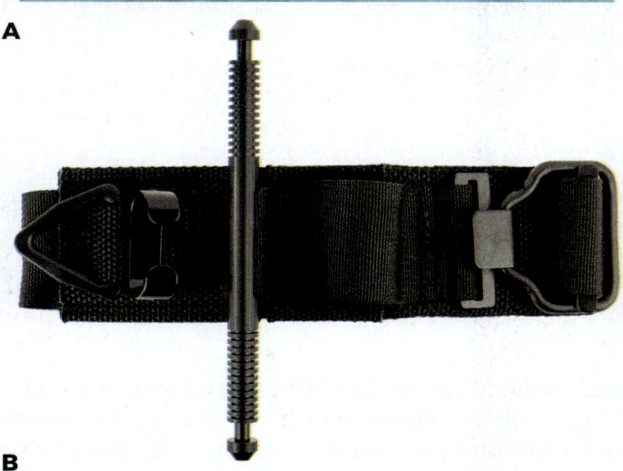

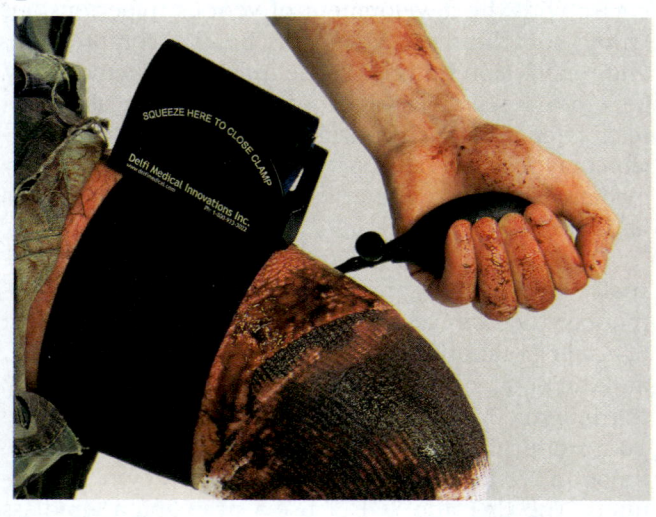

Figure 6-1 **A.** CAT. **B.** SOFTT. **C.** Emergency and Military Tourniquet.

A: Courtesy of Peter T. Pons, MD, FACEP; **B:** Courtesy of TacMed Solutions; **C:** Reproduced with permission from Emergency & Military Tourniquet, Delfi Medical, Retrieved from http://www.delfimedical.com/emergency-military-tourniquet/.

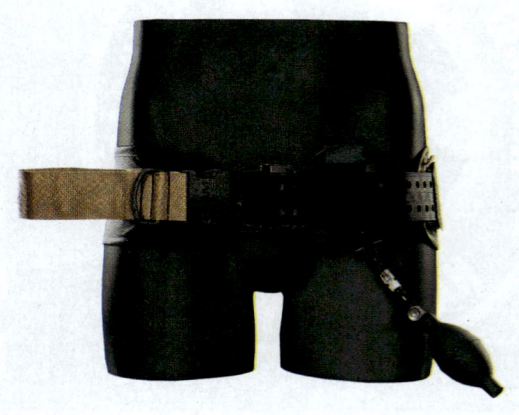

Figure 6-2 Junctional tourniquets have been used by the U.S. military in combat theaters to control severe bleeding.
Used with permission from SAM Medical.

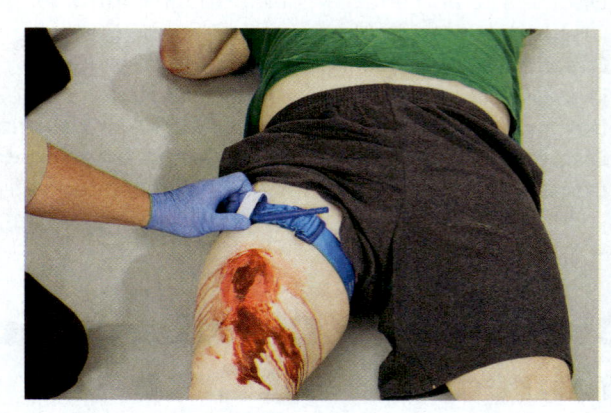

Figure 6-3 A tourniquet should be applied "high and tight," or as close to the junctional inguinal or axillae areas as possible unless a very prolonged field time is anticipated (significantly greater than two hours).
© Jones & Bartlett Learning. Photographed by Darren Stahlman.

a regular tourniquet cannot be applied (**Figure 6-2**). The Combat Ready Clamp (CRoC) was specifically designed for difficult inguinal bleeding during combat and works by compressing the femoral artery in the inguinal or groin area. The device is collapsible and lightweight and has a rounded plastic disk to apply direct pressure over the femoral artery. A safety strap is attached to the device to hold it around the torso.

Tourniquet Application

A tourniquet applied during direct threat care/hot zone should be "high and tight," or as close to the junctional inguinal or axillae areas as possible (**Figure 6-3**). During the indirect threat care/warm zone phase, tourniquets may be inspected and placed just proximal to the hemorrhaging wound if it is anticipated that the casualty will experience an extremely prolonged time prior to arrival at the receiving hospital. If one tourniquet does not completely stop the hemorrhage, then another one should be applied just proximal to the first. By placing two tourniquets side by side, the area of compression is doubled and the likelihood of successful control of hemorrhage may be increased. Once applied, the tourniquet site should not be covered; this allows it to be easily seen and monitored for recurrent hemorrhage. A tourniquet should be applied to any partial or total amputation, regardless of bleeding.

Application Tightness

A tourniquet should be applied tightly enough to block arterial flow and occlude the distal pulse. A device that only occludes venous outflow from a limb may actually increase hemorrhage from a wound. Furthermore, venous pooling from blood entering the extremity but not being able to exit could theoretically lead to compartment syndrome, which would require surgical intervention. A direct relationship exists between the amount of pressure required to control hemorrhage and the size of the limb. Thus, on average, a tourniquet will need to be placed more tightly on a leg to achieve hemorrhage control than on an arm. If a tourniquet is properly applied and bleeding is not successfully controlled, a second tourniquet may be used and placed immediately adjacent to the first. The addition of a second tourniquet provides additional compression and is usually successful in stopping bleeding in those cases where one device has proven inadequate.

Time Limit

Arterial tourniquets have been used routinely and very safely for up to 120 to 150 minutes in the operating room without significant nerve or muscle damage. Even in suburban or rural settings, most emergency medical services (EMS) transport times are significantly less than this period. In general, a tourniquet placed in the prehospital setting should remain in place until the patient reaches definitive care at the closest appropriate hospital. U.S. military use has not shown significant deterioration with prolonged application times. If application of a tourniquet is required, the patient has a high chance of needing emergency surgery to control hemorrhage. Thus, the ideal receiving facility for such a patient is a designated trauma center.

In the past, it was often recommended that a tourniquet be loosened every 10 to 15 minutes in order to allow for some blood flow back into the injured extremity with the assumption that this blood flow would help preserve the limb and prevent subsequent amputation. This practice only serves to increase the blood loss sustained by the patient and does nothing for the limb. Once applied, the tourniquet should be left in place until removed in the emergency department.

Expose and clearly mark tourniquets with the time of application, reapplication (as needed), and/or removal. If available, use a permanent marker to document time on the tourniquet. Tourniquet application should also be noted on the triage tag and/or patient care report. A tourniquet can be painful for a conscious patient to tolerate, and pain management should be considered, provided that the patient does not have signs of Class III or IV shock.

> ### BOX 6-1
> **Protocol for Tourniquet Application**
>
> Tourniquets should be used if controlling the hemorrhage with direct pressure or pressure dressing is not possible or fails. The steps in applying a tourniquet are as follows:
>
> 1. Apply a commercially manufactured tourniquet to the extremity at the level of the groin for the lower extremity or the axilla for the upper extremity.
> 2. Tighten the tourniquet until hemorrhage ceases and pulses are no longer palpable, and then secure it in place.
> 3. Write the time of tourniquet application on a piece of tape and secure it to the tourniquet. For example, "TK 2145" indicates that the tourniquet was applied at 2145 hours.
> 4. Leave the tourniquet uncovered so the site can be seen and monitored. If bleeding continues after application and tightening of the initial tourniquet, a second tourniquet can be applied immediately adjacent to the first.
> 5. Anticipate the need for pain management.
> 6. Transport the patient, ideally to a facility that has surgical capability.

> ### CHECK YOUR KNOWLEDGE
> **Insufficient tourniquet compression will:**
> a. increase the rate of sepsis in the damaged limb.
> b. generate circulatory embolisms.
> c. cause loss of blood to the general circulation.
> d. postpone the onset of shock.

Pelvic Binders

The New Brunswick Trauma Program Consensus Statement on Pelvic Binders notes that "... the circumferential compression obtained from a pelvic binder provides early stabilization for the patient who has suspected or confirmed unstable pelvic fracture. Stabilization of the pelvis reduces pelvic volume, which tamponades bleeding. It also reduces fracture movement, which reduces pain and helps reduce the risk of shearing major blood vessels during transport."

Stabilization of Pelvic Fractures

The 2016 TCCC Guidelines Change 1602 reported the results of the application of pelvic binders on traumatic injuries in human cadavers. "Commercial devices . . . and circumferential sheeting were compared in various combinations in five separate studies. All devices tested were found to provide near-anatomic fracture reduction with minimal overreduction. Angular motion was controlled during simulated patient care maneuvers in one study. In general, no significant difference was detected between the various commercial devices and circumferential sheet."

Further, the 2016 TCCC Guidelines Change 1602 cautions providers that "Placement of the binder at the level of the pubic symphysis and greater trochanters (*not* up by the iliac wings) was shown to reduce the unstable pelvic fracture most effectively with the least amount of force. Use caution not to place pelvic binder too high, which might result in inadequate reduction of the pelvic fracture and possibly increased bleeding."

Control of Pelvic Hemorrhage

Suspected high-energy pelvic fractures should have a binder applied in the field. While it is often not possible to differentiate a stable from an unstable fracture, a prudent TECC caregiver will apply a binder.

Several clinical studies have attempted to assess the effectiveness of the pelvic binder application on hemorrhage control. Fu and Wang conducted a retrospective review of 585 patients with pelvic fractures requiring transfer to a trauma center. Patients who had a pelvic binder applied before transfer spent less time in the hospital and needed fewer blood transfusions.

There is weak clinical evidence that pelvic binders application may reduce blood transfusion and lethal hemorrhage compared to other methods.

Indications and Contraindications for Pelvic Binder Use

After careful study, the Co-TCCC concluded "The indications selected for pelvic binder placement include suspected pelvic fracture based on a mechanism of severe blunt force or blast injury with one or more of the following indications:

- Pelvic pain
- Any major lower limb amputation or near amputation
- Physical examination findings suggestive of a pelvic fracture

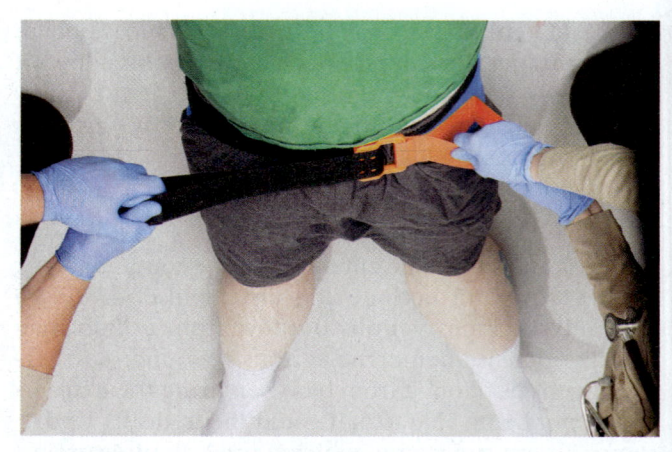

Figure 6-4 A commercially available pelvic binder.
© Jones & Bartlett Learning. Photographed by Darren Stahlman.

- Unconsciousness
- Shock"

The pelvic binder is contraindicated when there is an impaled object that would be covered by it. According to a 2017 statement by the New Brunswick Trauma Program, "In cases where the patient may have both fractured femur(s) and pelvic instability, the immobilization of the pelvis should be completed before immobilization of the femur(s), keeping in mind that traction splints interfere with use of the pelvic binder—using standard immobilization of lower extremities is recommended in these cases." Note that traction splint application is contraindicated if the casualty is hemodynamically unstable—expedite patient transport in these situations.

Application of Pelvic Binder

TCCC curricula caution providers not to logroll casualties with suspected pelvic fractures, as this may increase internal bleeding. Follow the manufacturer's directions and local protocols (**Figure 6-4**). Furthermore, the SAM junctional tourniquet and the Junctional Emergency Treatment Tool (JETT) may be used as improvised pelvic binders.

Shock Assessment

Shock is a state of change in cellular function from aerobic metabolism to anaerobic metabolism secondary to hypoperfusion of the tissue cells. As a result, the delivery of oxygen at the cellular level is inadequate to meet the body's metabolic needs. Shock is not defined as low blood pressure, rapid pulse rates, or cool, clammy skin; these are merely systemic manifestations of the entire pathologic process called shock. The correct definition of shock is a lack of tissue perfusion (oxygenation) at the cellular level that leads to anaerobic metabolism and impairment of energy production needed to support life.

Shock can kill a patient in the field. Although actual death may be delayed for several hours to several days or even weeks, the most common cause of that death is the failure of early resuscitation. The lack of perfusion of cells by oxygenated blood results in anaerobic metabolism and decreased function of cells needed for organ survival. Even when some cells are initially spared, death can occur later, because the remaining cells are unable to adequately carry out the function of that organ indefinitely (**Table 6-1**).

The prime determinants of cellular perfusion are the heart (acting as the pump, or the motor, of the system), fluid volume (acting as the hydraulic fluid), the blood vessels (serving as the conduits or plumbing), and, finally, the cells of the body. Based on these components of the perfusion system, shock may be classified into the following categories:

1. Hypovolemic shock is primarily hemorrhagic in the trauma patient and is related to loss of circulating blood cells with oxygen-carrying capacity and fluid volume. This is the most common cause of shock in the trauma patient.
2. Distributive (or vasogenic) shock is related to abnormality in vascular tone arising from several different causes. In trauma, the most common cause is spinal cord injury.
3. Cardiogenic shock is related to interference with the pump action of the heart.

By far the most common cause of shock in the trauma patient is hemorrhage, and the safest approach in managing the trauma patient in shock is to consider that the cause of the shock is hemorrhage until proven otherwise (**Table 6-2**).

Table 6-1 Organ Tolerance to Ischemia

Organ	Warm Ischemia Time
Heart, brain, lungs	4 to 6 minutes
Kidneys, liver, gastrointestinal tract	45 to 90 minutes
Muscle, bone, skin	4 to 6 hours

© National Association of Emergency Medical Technicians (NAEMT)

> **CHECK YOUR KNOWLEDGE**
>
> **Shock is defined as:**
>
> a. pulse rate at more than 140 beats per minute.
> b. inadequate tissue perfusion at the cellular level.
> c. diastolic blood pressure of less than 50 mm Hg for more than 20 minutes.
> d. pulse-oximeter Spo_2 reading of less than 84%.

Table 6-2 Types of Traumatic Shock

	Hypovolemic Shock	Cardiogenic Shock	Distributive Shock
Occurs in/due to	Loss of circulating volume	Impaired cardiac function	Abnormal dilation of the vascular compartment
	Blood loss (hemorrhagic shock) Plasma loss (burn patients)	Tension pneumothorax Pericardial tamponade Cardiac contusion	High spinal cord injury
Skin temperature/quality	Cool, clammy	Cool, clammy	Warm, dry
Skin color	Pale, cyanotic	Pale, cyanotic	Pink
Blood pressure	Drops	Drops	Drops
Level of consciousness	Altered	Altered	Lucid
Capillary refill time	Slowed	Slowed	Normal

© National Association of Emergency Medical Technicians (NAEMT)

Hypovolemic Shock

Acute loss of blood volume from hemorrhage (loss of plasma and RBCs) causes an imbalance in the relationship of fluid volume to the size of the container. The container retains its normal size, but the fluid volume is decreased. Hypovolemic shock is the most common cause of shock encountered in the TECC environment, and blood loss is by far the most common cause of shock in trauma patients.

When blood is lost from the circulation, the heart is stimulated to increase cardiac output by increasing the strength and rate of contractions. This stimulus results from the release of epinephrine from the adrenal glands. At the same time, the sympathetic nervous system releases norepinephrine to constrict blood vessels to reduce the size of the container and bring it more into proportion with the volume of remaining fluid. Vasoconstriction results in closing of the peripheral capillaries, which reduces oxygen delivery to those affected cells and forces the switch from aerobic to anaerobic metabolism at the cellular level.

These compensatory defense mechanisms work well up to a point and will help maintain the patient's vital signs for a period of time. A patient who has signs of compensation such as tachycardia is already in shock, not "going into shock." When the defense mechanisms can no longer compensate for the amount of blood lost, a patient's blood pressure will drop. This decrease in blood pressure marks the switch from compensated to decompensated shock—a sign of impending death. Unless aggressive resuscitation occurs, the patient who enters decompensated shock has only one more stage of decline left—irreversible shock, leading to death.

> **CHECK YOUR KNOWLEDGE**
>
> How is the transition from compensated to decompensated hypovolemic shock identified?
>
> a. Blood pressure drops.
> b. Pulse rate drops below 50 beats per minute.
> c. Patient starts to sweat copiously.
> d. Patient starts a run of vigorous, unproductive coughing.

Hemorrhagic Shock

The average 70-kg (150-lb) adult human has approximately 5 liters of circulating blood volume (**Figure 6-5**). Hemorrhagic shock (hypovolemic shock resulting from blood loss) is categorized into four classes, depending on the severity and amount of hemorrhage (**Table 6-3**), with the proviso that the values and descriptions for the criteria listed for these classes of shock should not be interpreted as absolute determinants of the class of shock, as significant overlap exists.

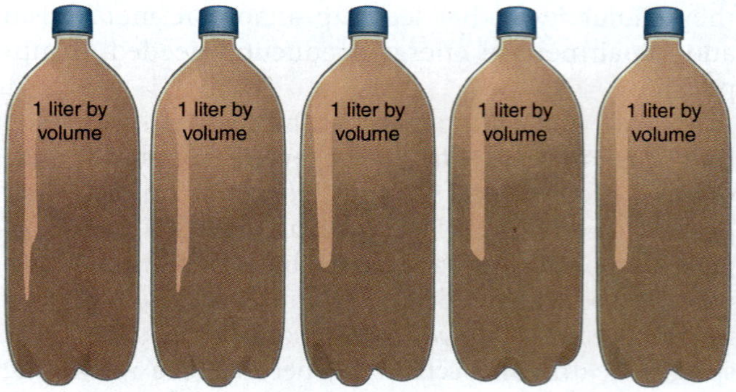

Figure 6-5 The average 70-kg (150-lb) adult human has approximately 5 liters of circulating blood volume.
© Jones & Bartlett Learning.

Class I hemorrhage represents a loss of up to 15% of blood volume in the adult (up to 750 milliliters [ml]) (**Figure 6-6**). This stage has few clinical manifestations. Tachycardia is often minimal, and no measurable changes in blood pressure, pulse, pressure, or ventilatory rate occur. Most healthy patients sustaining this amount of hemorrhage require only maintenance fluid as long as no further blood loss occurs. The body's compensatory mechanisms restore the intravascular container–fluid volume ratio and assist in the maintenance of blood pressure.

Class II hemorrhage represents a loss of 15% to 30% of blood volume (750 to 1,500 ml) (**Figure 6-7**). Most adults are capable of compensating for this amount of blood loss by activation of the sympathetic nervous system, which will maintain their blood pressure. Clinical findings include increased ventilatory rate, tachycardia, and a narrowed pulse pressure. The clinical clues to this phase are tachycardia, tachypnea, and normal systolic blood pressure. Because the blood pressure is normal, this is "compensated shock"—that is, the patient is in shock but is able to compensate for the time being. The patient often demonstrates anxiety or a flight response. Although not usually measured in the field, urine output drops slightly to between 20 and 30 ml/hour in an adult in an effort to preserve fluid. On occasion, these patients may require blood transfusion in the hospital; however, most will respond well to crystalloid infusion if hemorrhage is controlled at this point. These patients are often mildly anxious and diaphoretic.

Class III hemorrhage represents a loss of 30% to 40% of blood volume (1,500 to 2,000 ml) (**Figure 6-8**).

LESSON 6 Indirect Threat Care/Warm Zone: MARCH—Circulation

Table 6-3 Classification of Hemorrhagic Shock

	Class I	Class II	Class III	Class IV
Blood loss (ml)	<750	750–1,500	1,500–2,000	>2,000
Blood loss (% blood volume)	<15%	15–30%	30–40%	>40%
Pulse rate	<100	100–120	120–140	>140
Blood pressure	Normal	Normal	Decreased	Decreased
Pulse pressure (mm Hg)	Normal or increased	Decreased	Decreased	Decreased
Ventilatory rate	14–20	20–30	30–40	>35
Central nervous system/mental status	Slightly anxious	Mildly anxious	Anxious, confused	Confused, lethargic
Fluid replacement	Crystalloid	Crystalloid	Crystalloid and blood	Crystalloid and blood

Note: The values and descriptions for the criteria listed for these classes of shock should not be interpreted as absolute determinants of the class of shock, as significant overlap exists.

Source: From American College of Surgeons (ACS) Committee on Trauma. *Advanced Trauma Life Support for Doctors: Student Course Manual*. 8th ed. Chicago, IL: ACS; 2008.

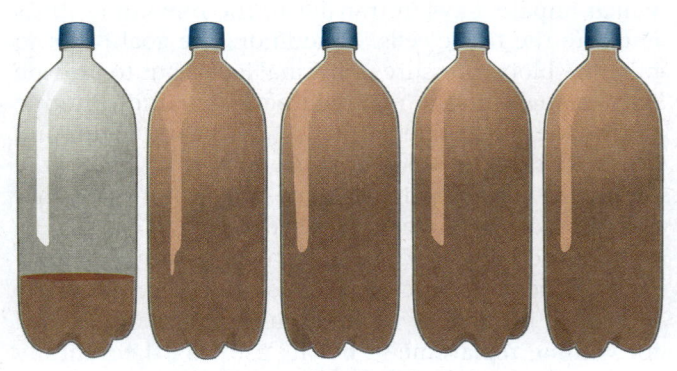

750 ml blood loss / 4.25 liters blood volume
Class I hemorrhage = blood loss up to 750 ml

Figure 6-6 Class I hemorrhage.
© Jones & Bartlett Learning.

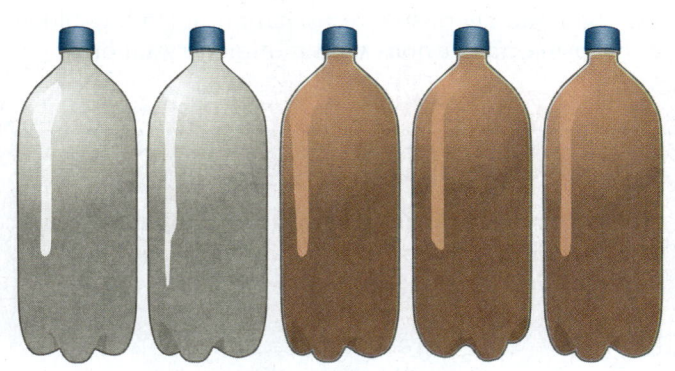

2000 ml blood loss / 3.0 liters blood volume
Class III hemorrhage = blood loss up to 2,000 ml

Figure 6-8 Class III hemorrhage.
© Jones & Bartlett Learning.

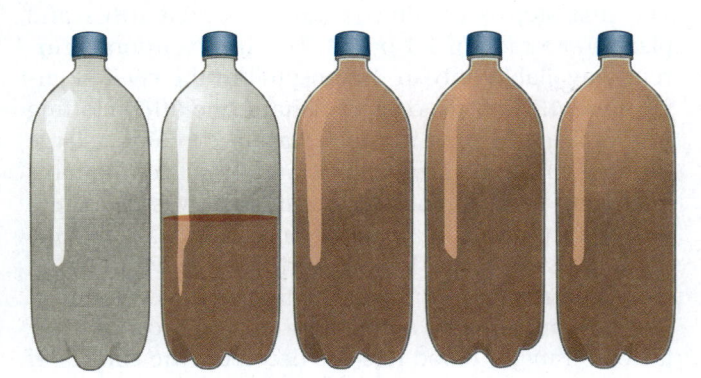

1500 ml blood loss / 3.5 liters blood volume
Class II hemorrhage = blood loss up to 1,500 ml

Figure 6-7 Class II hemorrhage.
© Jones & Bartlett Learning.

When blood loss reaches this point, most patients are no longer able to compensate for the volume loss, and hypotension occurs. The classic findings of shock are obvious and include tachycardia (heart rate greater than 120 beats/minute), tachypnea (ventilatory rate of 30 to 40 breaths/minute), and severe anxiety or confusion. Urine output falls to 5 to 15 ml/hour. Many of these patients will require blood transfusion and surgical intervention for adequate resuscitation and control of hemorrhage.

Class IV hemorrhage represents a loss of more than 40% of blood volume (greater than 2,000 ml) (**Figure 6-9**). This stage of severe shock is characterized by marked tachycardia (heart rate greater than

Figure 6-9 Class IV hemorrhage.
2500 ml blood loss / 2.5 liters blood volume
Class IV hemorrhage = greater than 2,000 ml
© Jones & Bartlett Learning.

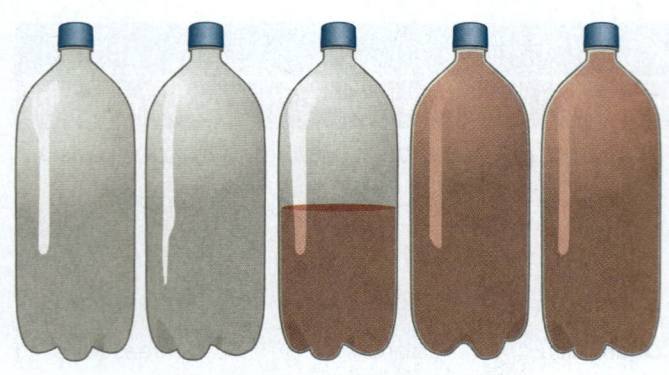

140 beats/minute), tachypnea (ventilatory rate greater than 35 breaths/minute), profound confusion or lethargy, and greatly decreased systolic blood pressure, typically in the range of 60 mm Hg. These patients truly have only minutes to live. Survival depends on immediate control of hemorrhage (surgery for internal hemorrhage) and aggressive resuscitation, including blood and plasma transfusions with minimal crystalloid.

> **CHECK YOUR KNOWLEDGE**
>
> The sympathetic nervous system is capable of handling a Class _____ hemorrhage situation.
>
> a. II
> b. III
> c. IV
> d. The sympathetic nervous system is incapable of handling a hemorrhage situation.

Fluid Resuscitation of Hemorrhagic Shock

The rapidity with which a patient develops shock depends on how fast blood is lost from the circulation. A trauma patient who has lost blood needs to have the source of blood loss stopped, and, if significant blood loss has occurred, blood replacement needs to be accomplished. The fluid that has been lost is whole blood—containing all of its various components, including RBCs with oxygen-carrying capacity, clotting factors, and proteins to maintain oncotic pressure.

Whole blood replacement, or even component therapy, may not be available in the tactical prehospital environment. TECC caregivers must take measures to control external blood loss, provide minimal intravenous (IV) electrolyte solution (plasma when available), and transport rapidly to a hospital trauma center, where blood, plasma, and clotting factors are available and emergent operative steps to control blood loss can be performed, as necessary.

Shock research has demonstrated that for lost blood, the replacement ratio with electrolyte solution should be 3 liters of replacement for each liter of blood lost. This high ratio of replacement fluid is required because only about one-fourth to one-third of the volume of an isotonic crystalloid solution such as normal saline (NS) or lactated Ringer solution remains in the intravascular space 30 to 60 minutes after infusing it.

Shock research has also shown that the administration of a limited volume of electrolyte solution before blood replacement is the safest approach while transporting to the hospital. The result of administering too much crystalloid is increased interstitial fluid (edema), which impairs oxygen transfer to the remaining RBCs and into the tissue cells. In addition, the goal is not to raise the blood pressure to normal levels but to provide only enough fluid to maintain perfusion and continue to provide oxygenated RBCs to the heart, brain, and lungs. Raising the blood pressure to normal levels only serves to dilute clotting factors, disrupt any clot that has formed, and increase hemorrhage.

The best crystalloid solution for treating hemorrhagic shock is lactated Ringer solution. Normal saline is another isotonic crystalloid solution that can be used for volume replacement, but its use may theoretically produce hyperchloremia (marked increase in the blood chloride level), leading to acidosis.

With significant blood loss, the optimal replacement fluid is ideally as near to whole blood as possible. The first step is administration of packed RBCs and plasma at a ratio of 1:1 or 1:2. This intervention is currently available only in the hospital in the civilian environment. Platelets, cryoprecipitate, and other clotting factors are added as needed. Plasma contains a large number of the clotting factors and other components needed to control blood loss from small vessels. There are 13 factors in the coagulation cascade. In patients with massive blood loss requiring large volumes of blood replacement, most of the factors have been lost. Plasma transfusion is a reliable source of most of these factors. If major blood loss has occurred, the control of hemorrhage from large vessels by operative management or, in some cases, endovascular placement of coils or clotting sponges is the priority.

> **CHECK YOUR KNOWLEDGE**
>
> **What is the goal in fluid resuscitation of hemorrhagic shock?**
>
> a. Aggressively administer crystalloid solutions to get systolic blood pressure to 120 mm Hg.
> b. Alternate between crystalloid and plasma administrations to avoid cavitation.
> c. Alternate between Ringer lactate and saline to smooth out electrolyte imbalance.
> d. Provide just enough fluid to maintain perfusion and continue to provide oxygenated RBCs to the heart, brain, and lungs.

Neurogenic Shock

Neurogenic "shock," or more appropriately neurogenic hypotension, occurs when a spinal cord injury interrupts the sympathetic nervous system pathway. This usually involves injury to the lower cervical, thoracolumbar, and thoracic levels. Because of the loss of sympathetic control of the vascular system, which controls the smooth muscles in the walls of the blood vessels, the peripheral vessels dilate below the level of injury. The marked decrease in systemic vascular resistance and peripheral vasodilation that occurs as the container for the blood volume increases results in relative hypovolemia. The patient is not really hypovolemic, but the normal blood volume insufficiently fills an expanded container.

Tissue oxygenation usually remains adequate in the neurogenic form of shock, and blood flow remains normal although the blood pressure is low (neurogenic hypotension). In addition, energy production remains adequate in neurogenic hypotension. Therefore, this decrease in blood pressure is not shock because energy production remains unaffected. However, because there is less resistance to blood flow, the systolic and diastolic pressures are lower (**Table 6-4**).

Decompensated hypovolemic shock and neurogenic shock both produce a decreased systolic blood pressure. However, the other vital and clinical signs, as well as the treatment for each, are different. Decreased systolic and diastolic pressures and a narrow pulse pressure characterize hypovolemic shock. Neurogenic shock also displays decreased systolic and diastolic pressures, but the pulse pressure remains normal or is widened. Hypovolemia produces cold, clammy, pale, or cyanotic skin and delayed capillary refilling time. In neurogenic shock the patient has warm, dry skin, especially below the area of injury. The pulse in hypovolemic shock patients is weak, thready, and rapid. In neurogenic shock, because of unopposed parasympathetic activity on the heart, bradycardia is typically seen rather than tachycardia, but the pulse quality may be weak. Hypovolemia produces a decreased level of consciousness, or at least anxiety, and often combativeness. In the absence of a traumatic brain injury the patient with neurogenic shock is usually alert, oriented, and lucid when in the supine position.

> **BOX 6-2**
>
> **Neurogenic Shock Versus Spinal Shock**
>
> The term *neurogenic shock* refers to a disruption of the sympathetic nervous system, typically from injury to the spinal cord or a hemodynamic phenomenon, which results in significant dilation of the peripheral arteries. If untreated, this may result in impaired perfusion to the body's tissues. Although typically lumped together, this condition should not be confused with spinal shock, a term that refers to a temporary decrease in the function of reflex arcs within the spinal cord that occurs in conjunction with spinal cord injury.

Table 6-4 Signs Associated With Types of Shock

Vital Sign	Hypovolemic	Neurogenic	Cardiogenic
Skin temperature/quality	Cool, clammy	Warm, dry	Cool, clammy
Skin color	Pale, cyanotic	Pink	Pale, cyanotic
Blood pressure	Drops	Drops	Drops
Level of consciousness	Altered	Lucid	Altered
Capillary refilling time	Slowed	Normal	Slowed

© National Association of Emergency Medical Technicians (NAEMT)

Patients with neurogenic shock frequently have associated injuries that produce significant hemorrhage. Therefore, a patient who has neurogenic shock and signs of hypovolemia, such as tachycardia, should be treated as if blood loss is present.

> **CHECK YOUR KNOWLEDGE**
>
> **Narrow pulse pressure distinguishes _____ shock from _____ shock.**
> a. hemorrhagic; pulmonary
> b. hypovolemic; neurogenic
> c. neurogenic; cardiogenic
> d. neurogenic; pulmonary

Intravenous Access

Another important step in resuscitation is the restoration of the cardiovascular system to an adequate perfusing volume as quickly as possible. This step does not involve restoring blood pressure to normal but rather providing enough fluid to ensure that vital organs are being perfused. Because blood is usually not available in the prehospital setting, lactated Ringer or another isotonic crystalloid solution such as normal saline is used for trauma resuscitation. In addition to sodium and chloride, lactated Ringer solution contains small amounts of potassium, calcium, and lactate and is an effective volume expander. Crystalloid solutions, such as lactated Ringer and NS, however, do not replace the oxygen-carrying capacity of the lost RBCs or the lost platelets that are necessary for clotting and bleeding control. Therefore, rapid transport of a severely injured patient to an appropriate facility is an absolute necessity.

Within the indirect threat care/warm zone a single 18-gauge catheter is recommended. It provides adequate access for delivery of resuscitation fluids and medications. Until the patient is out of the tactical area, a saline lock is recommended over an IV line, unless fluids are immediately needed. Flush the saline lock with 5 ml NS immediately and repeat every 1 to 2 hours to keep the line open. Note that an IV line should not be attempted on an extremity that has a significant wound proximal to the IV insertion site.

Intraosseous Access

If the patient is in the indirect threat/warm zone and needs fluid resuscitation, or if IV access cannot be obtained, intraosseous (IO) access may be appropriate. This method of vascular access can be accomplished in a number of ways. It can be established via the sternal technique, using appropriately designed devices (**Figure 6-10**).

Specially designed devices such as the Pyng FAST1, the Bone Injection Gun, and the EZ-IO may also be used to establish access through sites in the distal tibia above the ankle, the proximal tibia, the distal femur, the proximal humerus, or the sternum (though an EZ-IO should not be used at the sternal site) (**Figure 6-11**).

For delayed or prolonged transport to definitive care, IO vascular access may have a role in adult trauma patients.

Intraosseous Procedure

This technique may be performed in both adult and pediatric patients, using a variety of commercially available devices.

1. Assemble the equipment, which includes IO infusion needle, syringe filled with at least 5 ml of sterile saline, antiseptic, IV fluid and tubing, and tape. Ensure proper body substance isolation. Place the patient in a supine position. The choice of insertion site may be the humeral head, distal femur, tibia, or sternum. For pediatric patients, a common insertion

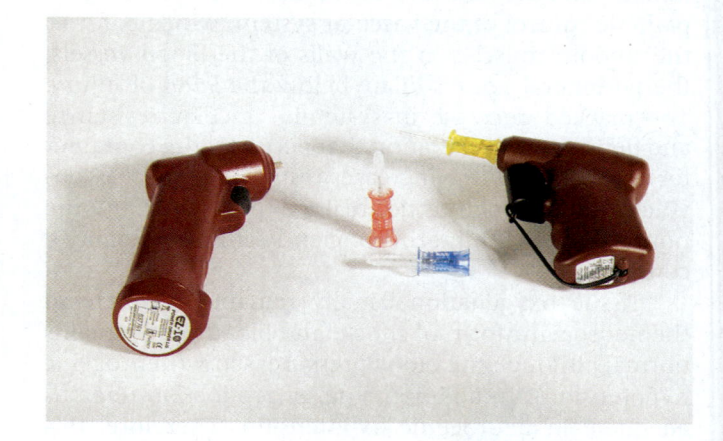

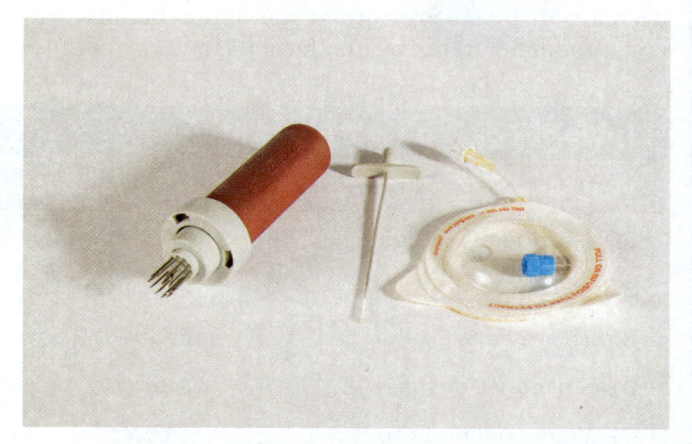

Figure 6-10 **A.** IO needles and IO gun for manual insertion (various sizes shown). **B.** IO sternal driver.

© Jones & Bartlett Learning. Photographed by Darren Stahlman.

site is the anterior-medial proximal tibia just below the tibial tuberosity. The prehospital care provider identifies the tibia is the insertion site; the lower extremity is stabilized by another provider. Clean the insertion site area with an antiseptic (**Figure 6-12**).
2. Holding the drill and needle at a 90-degree angle to the selected bone, activate the drill and insert the rotating needle through the skin and into the bone cortex. A "pop" will be felt upon entering the bone cortex (**Figure 6-13**).
3. When you feel a lack of resistance against the needle, release the trigger of the drill. While holding the needle, remove the drill from the needle (**Figure 6-14**).
4. Release and remove the trocar from the center of the needle (**Figure 6-15**).

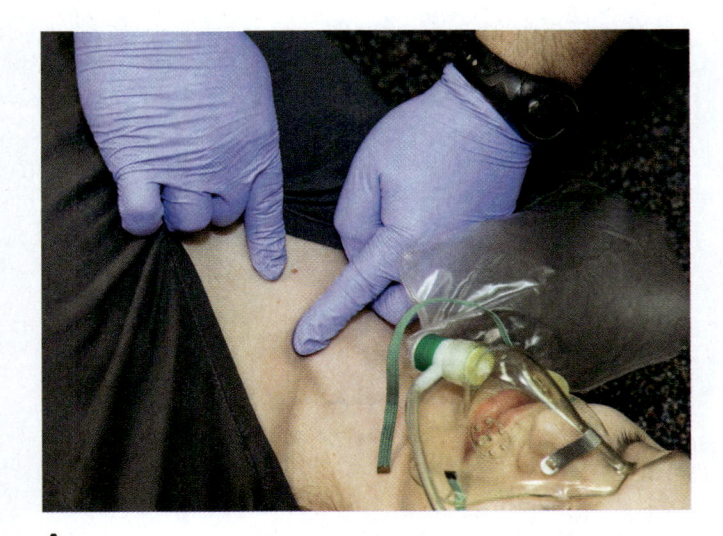

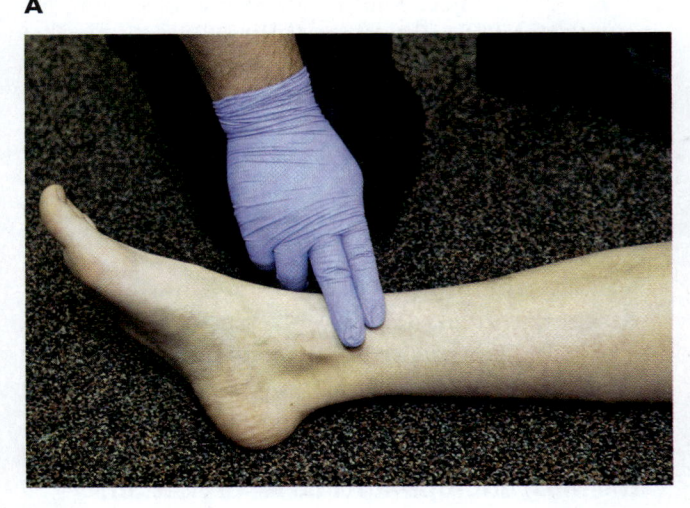

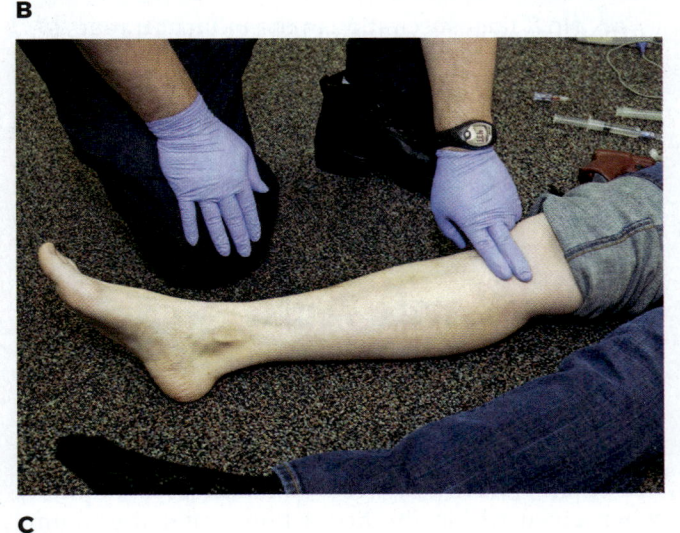

Figure 6-11 **A.** Sternal insertion site in the manubrium below the suprasternal notch. Note that the EZ-IO device cannot be used at the sternal site. **B.** Distal tibial insertion site above the ankle. **C.** Proximal tibial insertion site below the knee.
© National Association of Emergency Medical Technicians (NAEMT).

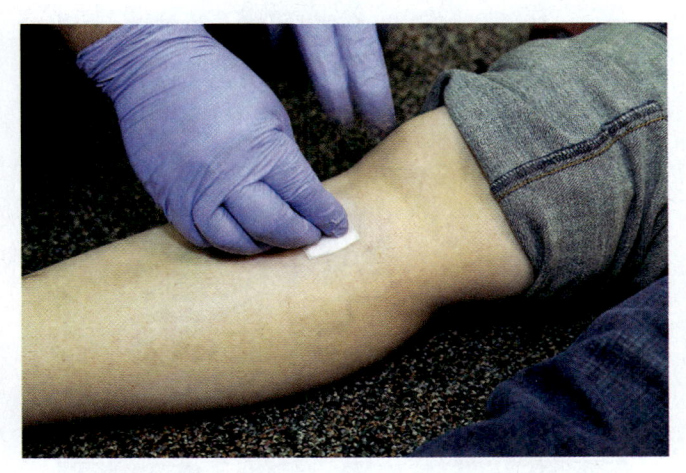

Figure 6-12 The insertion site area is cleaned with an antiseptic.
© National Association of Emergency Medical Technicians (NAEMT).

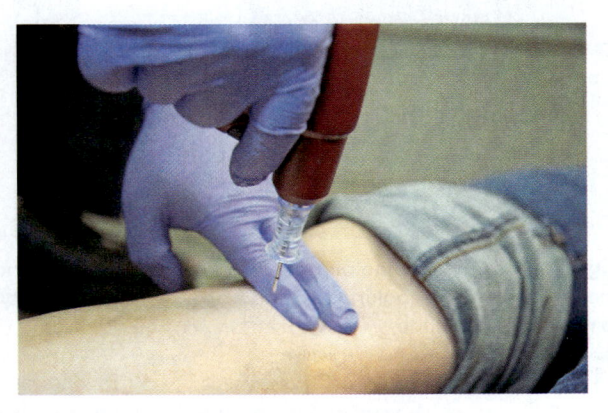

Figure 6-13 The drill and needle are held at a 90-degree angle to the selected bone, the drill is activated, and the rotating needle is inserted through the skin and into the bone cortex.
© National Association of Emergency Medical Technicians (NAEMT).

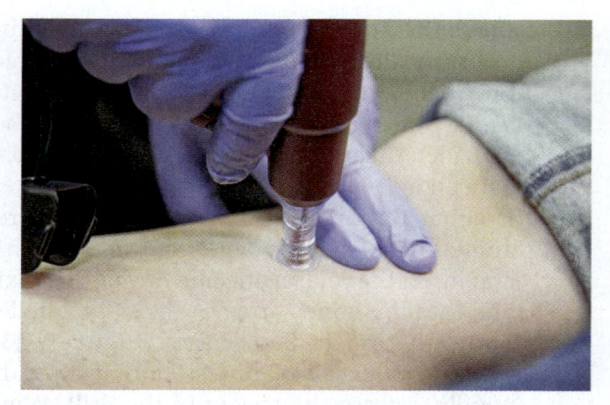

Figure 6-14 When a lack of resistance is felt against the needle, the trigger of the drill is released.
© National Association of Emergency Medical Technicians (NAEMT).

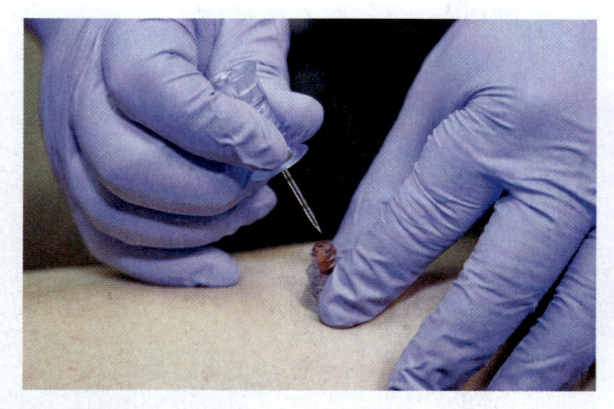

Figure 6-15 The trocar is removed from the center of the needle.
© National Association of Emergency Medical Technicians (NAEMT).

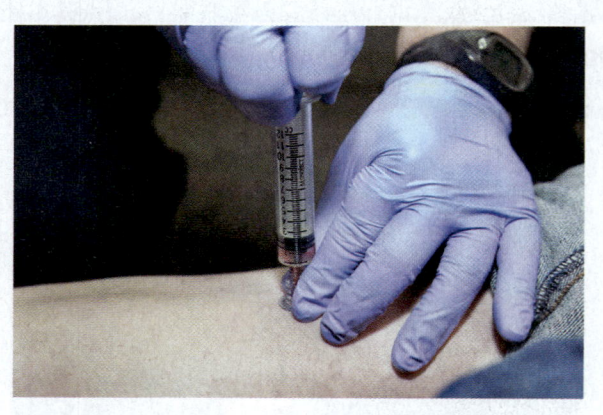

Figure 6-16 The syringe plunger is drawn back slightly, and the EMS provider is looking for fluid from the marrow cavity to mix with the saline.
© National Association of Emergency Medical Technicians (NAEMT).

5. Attach the syringe with saline to the needle hub. Draw back with the syringe plunger slightly, looking for fluid from the marrow cavity to mix with the saline. "Dry" taps are not uncommon (**Figure 6-16**).

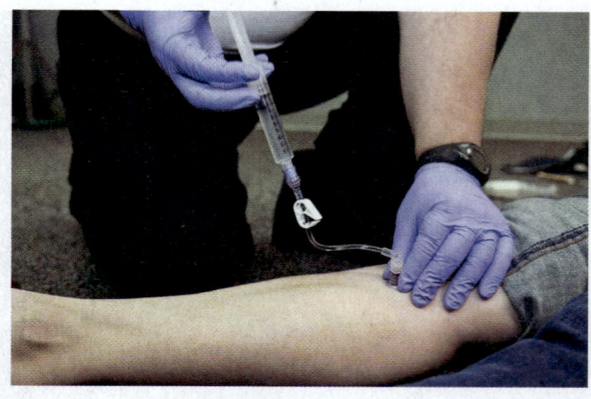

Figure 6-17 Five ml of saline is injected.
© National Association of Emergency Medical Technicians (NAEMT).

6. Next, inject 5 ml of the saline, observing for signs of infiltration. If there are no signs of infiltration, remove the syringe from the needle hub, attach the IV tubing, and set the flow rate. Secure the needle and IV tubing (**Figure 6-17**).

> **CHECK YOUR KNOWLEDGE**
>
> **You are treating a patient in the indirect threat care/warm zone who has a gunshot wound to the gut and a systolic blood pressure of 90 by palpation. There will be a 15- to 20-minute delay in moving the patient to the evacuation care/cold zone. What is the most appropriate fluid resuscitation?**
>
> a. No fluid resuscitation in the indirect threat care/warm zone
> b. 18-gauge needle with saline lock
> c. Intraosseous access and one IV line of a crystalloid solution
> d. Two 14-gauge IV lines flowing lactated Ringer

Tranexamic Acid

Tranexamic acid (TXA) is an effective antifibrinolytic that blocks the interaction of plasminogen with the lysine residues of fibrin. Administration of TXA to hemorrhage patients has had beneficial effects, including decreased transfusion need and decreased mortality when given within the first 3 hours after the trauma event. This performance was verified in the 2010 Clinical Randomization of an Antifibrinolytic in Significant Hemorrhage 2 (CRASH-2) study.

Another study published in 2012, Military Application of Tranexamic Acid in Trauma Emergency and

Resuscitation (MATTERs), examined 896 casualties treated at the Bastion Hospital in Afghanistan. Findings indicated that use of TXA with blood component–based resuscitation following combat injury resulted in improved measures of coagulopathy and survival.

TXA can be administered by mouth (Lysteda) or IV (Cyklokapron), or applied directly on bleeding. In the TECC arena TXA is used as an adjunct to treat patients in hemorrhagic shock. Contraindications include severe renal insufficiency and hematuria (blood in urine).

TXA Administration

Administration should be as soon as possible, but no later than 3 hours after wounding. TXA administration should be done per local protocols. The recommendations that follow describe the course of administration employed in the hospital and associated with the studies that have been published demonstrating efficacy in that arena.

Key information for administration is as follows:

- TXA is supplied in 1-gram (1,000 mg) ampules.
- Inject 1 gram (g) of TXA into a 100-ml bag of NS or lactated Ringer.
- Infuse slowly over 10 minutes.
- Rapid IV push may cause hypotension and gastric distress.
- If there is a new-onset drop in blood pressure during the infusion, *slow down* the TXA infusion.

Administer crystalloid or blood products per protocol. If the patient is still in the field and fluid resuscitation has been completed, a second dose of TXA may be authorized before the patient arrives at the trauma center. Follow the same protocol as the first dose.

> ### CHECK YOUR KNOWLEDGE
>
> **You are administering an IV dose of TXA and the patient complains of dizziness and vomits. You should:**
>
> a. speed up the rate of TXA infusion.
> b. slow down the rate of TXA infusion.
> c. stop IV administration of TXA.
> d. check patient blood pressure, and stop TXA if systolic is below 60 mm Hg.

Damage Control Resuscitation

In a 2017 paper on damage control resuscitation, Mizobata noted, ". . . damage control resuscitation (DCR), the strategic approach to the trauma patient who presents in extremis, consists of balanced resuscitation, hemostatic resuscitation, and prevention of acidosis, hypothermia, and hypocalcemia. In balanced resuscitation, fluid administration is restricted and hypotension is allowed until definitive hemostatic measures [can be instituted]. The administration of blood products consisting of fresh frozen plasma, packed red blood cells, and platelets, the ratio of which resembles whole blood, is recommended early in the resuscitation."

Coagulopathy and the "Lethal Triad"

Mizobata states: "Coagulopathy is a condition in which the blood's ability to coagulate (form clots) is impaired. This condition can cause a tendency toward prolonged or excessive bleeding, which may occur spontaneously or following an injury or medical and dental procedures. Traditionally, the coagulopathy observed in trauma patients was thought to be 'resuscitation-associated coagulopathy,' which is caused by the consumption of coagulation factors, dilution of coagulation factors after massive infusion, hypothermia, and acidosis. An increasing incidence of coagulopathy was observed with increasing amounts of intravenous fluids administered.

The administration of large amounts of fluids and blood products, exposure of the body, and surgical intervention performed for resuscitation cause the hypothermia. Alcohol and drugs, which are one of the causes of trauma incidents, increase heat loss from the trauma patient. Hypothermia is observed in about 60% of trauma patients who require emergency operative interventions. It is associated with an increased risk of bleeding and mortality of trauma patients. Inadequate tissue perfusion due to hemorrhagic shock results in anaerobic metabolism and the subsequent production of lactic acid, which causes metabolic acidosis. The high chloride content in crystalloid solutions, such as 0.9% normal saline, exacerbates the metabolic acidosis.

The term 'lethal triad' was used to describe the physiologic derangement observed in these patients and refers to the triad of the deteriorating status of acute coagulopathy, hypothermia, and acidosis of exsanguinating trauma patients. The lethal triad forms a downward spiral, and further hemorrhage deteriorates the triad.

Mizobata further states that: "DCR directly addresses the trauma-induced coagulopathy immediately upon patient admission or in the prehospital setting. DCR consists of balanced resuscitation, hemostatic resuscitation, and prevention of acidosis, hypothermia, and hypocalcemia."

TECC Damage Control Resuscitation

Working within the tactical arena, fluid administration should only be provided to patients experiencing hemorrhagic shock. The TECC caregiver can identify those casualties when they have a weak or absent radial pulse and are exhibiting an altered mental status without evidence of a head injury.

The amount of fluid administered should be limited. Excessive crystalloid fluid increases interstitial fluid, creating edema that could impair the transfer of oxygen with the remaining red blood cells and tissues. Your goal is not to raise the blood pressure to normal levels. A trauma patient filled with crystalloids to get to a normal blood pressure will experience diluted clotting factors, increasing coagulopathy, increased rate of hemorrhage, and will "blow-off" blood clots.

Traumatic Brain Injury

Traumatic brain injury (TBI) can occur either from direct contact to the head or when the brain is shaken within the skull, such as from a blast or whiplash during a car accident. In a brain injury, the person may experience a change in consciousness that can range from becoming disoriented and confused to coma. The person may also have a loss of memory for the time immediately before or after the event that caused the injury.

The severity of the TBI is determined at the time of the injury and is based on the length of the loss of consciousness, the length of either memory loss or disorientation, and how responsive the individual was after the injury. Not all injuries to the head result in a TBI, however.

The Department of Defense (DoD) estimates that 22% of all combat casualties from Iraq and Afghanistan sustained brain injuries. TBI is also a significant cause of disability outside of military settings, most often as the result of assaults, falls, automobile accidents, or sports injuries. TBI can involve symptoms ranging from headaches, irritability, and sleep disorders to memory problems, slower thinking, and depression.

Within the TECC arena, a TBI casualty could die from hypotension and hypoxia. Patients with a suspected TBI who also present with a weak or absent pulse need fluid resuscitation. The goal is to restore a normal radial pulse. If you have access to a blood pressure monitoring device, maintain a minimum systolic blood pressure of 90 mm Hg in the context of TBI.

> **CHECK YOUR KNOWLEDGE**
>
> **A casualty with signs of traumatic brain injury and hypotension:**
>
> a. is triaged as a gray/black tag patient.
> b. requires fluid resuscitation to maintain a normal radial pulse.
> c. must be hyperventilated with high-flow oxygen.
> d. needs to be transported in the Trendelenburg position.

Summary

- Apply tourniquets as necessary and assess existing tourniquets for adequacy of bleeding control and absence of distal pulses.
- Apply a pelvic binder for suspected pelvic fracture.
- The best indicators of shock in an indirect threat/warm zone are decreased level of consciousness and/or abnormal character of the radial pulse.
- The use of a single 18-gauge catheter is recommended for IV access.
- IO access can be an alternative to IV if the casualty requires fluid resuscitation or IV medications and IV access cannot be obtained.
- TXA has been shown to slow or stop some internal bleeding in trauma centers. It's efficacy in the prehospital setting remains controversial but is gaining in popularity.
- Fluid administration should be reserved for casualties experiencing hemorrhagic shock.

Skill Stations

Intraosseous Access

1. Use appropriate infection control precautions.
2. Gather and prepare equipment.
3. Identify at least two anatomic sites (adult and pediatric).
4. Identify and cleanse insertion site.
5. Ensure needle set and driver are seated.
6. Remove needle safety cap from device.
7. Position needle at a 90-degree angle to the bone.
8. Ensure needle rests against the bone with at least 5 mm of visible catheter.
9. Engage driver trigger and apply firm, steady, downward pressure until entering the medullary space (decreased resistance).
10. Hold the hub in place while removing power driver.

11. Remove stylet and confirm catheter stability.
12. Attach extension set to hub's Luer lock.
13. Aspirate blood/bone marrow for confirmation.
14. Flush with 10 ml of NS.
15. Stabilize and monitor site for signs of displacement and/or complications.
16. For responsive casualties, consider anesthetic agent.
17. Connect fluids and use pressure bag as needed.
18. To remove:
    - Attach syringe to EZ-IO catheter and remove by applying traction with clockwise twisting, taking care not to rock or bend the catheter.
    - Appropriately dispose of sharps.

IV Administration of TXA

1. Prepare and inspect equipment.
2. Initiate a ruggedized saline lock on the training device.
3. Explain the procedure to the casualty, and ask about known allergies.
4. On the simulated medication vial, confirm the correct dose of TXA: 1 g.
5. Attach a needle to the 10-ml syringe.
    a. Draw 10 ml of air into the 10-ml syringe.
    b. Clean the top of the TXA vial with an alcohol swab.
    c. Insert the needle into the TXA vial.
    d. Inject 5 ml of air into the TXA vial.
    e. Draw 5 ml of the TXA solution into the syringe.
    f. Inject 5 ml of air into the TXA vial.
    g. Draw the remaining 5 ml of TXA solution into the syringe.
6. Confirm that 1 g of TXA in 10 cc is now in the syringe.
7. Withdraw the needle from the TXA vial.
    a. Detach the needle from the syringe and discard it into the sharps container.
8. Attach a new needle to the syringe.
9. Clean the port on the mini-bag of NS with an alcohol swab.
10. Insert the needle into the port of the mini-bag of NS.
11. Inject the 10 ml of TXA solution into the mini-bag.
12. Withdraw the needle from the port of the mini-bag.
    a. Discard the needle and syringe into the sharps container.
13. Shake and knead the mini-bag to assure thorough mixing of the TXA.
14. Confirm 1 g of TXA is mixed in the 110 cc and is now in the mini-bag.
15. Clean the injection port on ruggedized saline lock.
16. Attach an IV administration set to the mini-bag of TXA.
    a. Connect the other end of the IV administration set to the saline lock.
17. Open the flow through the IV administration set.
18. Adjust the flow through the IV administration set to 18 gtt/10 sec (= 108 gtt/min = 10.8 ml/min = 108 ml/10 min). This rate will infuse 1 g of TXA in 110-ml volume in just over 10 minutes.
19. Observe the casualty for adverse side effects.
20. Detach and discard the IV administration set and mini-bag.
21. Document TXA administration.

REFERENCES AND RESOURCES

Fu CY, Wu YT, Liao CH, Kang SC, Wang SY, Hsu YP, Lin BC, Yuan KC, Kuo IM, Ouyang CH. Pelvic circumferential compression devices benefit patients with pelvic fractures who need transfers. *Am J Emerg Med.* 2013;31(10):1432-1436.

Mizobata Y. Damage control resuscitation: a practical approach for severely hemorrhagic patients and its effects on trauma surgery. *J Intensive Care.* 2017;5:4.

Morrison JJ, Dubose JJ, Rasmussen TE, Midwinter MJ. Military Application of Tranexamic Acid in Trauma Emergency Resuscitation (MATTERs) study. *Arch Surg.* 2012;147(2):113-119.

Napolitano LM. Prehospital tranexamic acid: what is the current evidence? *Trauma Surg Acute Care Open.* 2017;2(1):e000056.

National Association of Emergency Medical Technicians. *PHTLS: Prehospital Trauma Life Support.* 9th ed. Burlington, MA: Public Safety Group; 2019.

New Brunswick Trauma Program. NBTP Consensus Statement Pelvic Binders. 2017;1. https://nbtrauma.ca/wp-content/uploads/2018/02/FAQ-Pelvic-Binder-May-2017-final.pdf. Accessed February 20, 2019.

Roberts I, Shakur H, Coats T, Hunt B, Balogun E, Barnetson L, Cook L, Kawahara T, Perel P, Prieto-Merino D,

Ramos M, Cairns J, Guerriero C. The CRASH-2 trial: a randomised controlled trial and economic evaluation of the effects of tranexamic acid on death, vascular occlusive events and transfusion requirement in bleeding trauma patients. *Health Technol Assess*. 2013;17(10):1-79.

Scerbo MH, Mumm JP, Gates K, Love JD, Wade CE, Holcomb JB, Cotton BA. Safety and appropriateness of tourniquets in 105 civilians. *Prehosp Emerg Care*. 2016;20(6):712-722.

Shackelford S, Hammesfahr R, Morissette D, Montgomery HR, Kerr W, Broussard M, Bennett BL, Dorlac WC, Bree S, Butler FK. The use of pelvic binders in tactical combat casualty care: TCCC guidelines change 1602 7 November 2016. *J Spec Oper Med*. 2017;17(1):135-147.

Snyder D, Tsou A, Schoelles K. *Efficacy of Prehospital Application of Tourniquets and Hemostatic Dressings to Control Traumatic External Hemorrhage*. Washington, DC: National Highway Traffic Safety Administration; 2014.

LESSON 7

Indirect Threat Care/Warm Zone: Hypothermia and Head Injury

LESSON OBJECTIVES
- Understand the negative impact of hypothermia on a trauma patient.
- Describe current interventions for traumatic brain injury (TBI).
- Understand available monitoring devices and ways to reassess the patient.
- Discuss options in analgesic utilization.
- Describe fire used as a weapon.
- Review current burn care interventions.
- Discuss the importance of eye protection and eye injury intervention.
- Understand available evacuation devices and methods of effective patient communication.
- Discuss cardiopulmonary resuscitation (CPR) attempts in a multicasualty event.
- Discuss the importance of documentation.

Overview of Circulation in Indirect Threat Care/Warm Zone

Lesson 7: Indirect Threat Care/Warm Zone: Hypothermia and Head Injury wraps up indirect threat care/warm zone by looking at the balance of MARCH practices. Once bleeding control is completed, the tactical emergency casualty care (TECC) provider can look at the "H"—hypothermia and head injury. Remember that the tactical situation continues to be unpredictable and the indirect threat/warm zone could suddenly deteriorate into a direct threat/hot zone and require immediate movement of the patient and caregiver.

Hypothermia

Hypothermia is the third most serious condition in a trauma patient, ranking close to hypoxia and hypovolemia. It is generally considered a concerning sign, yet the actual temperature at which hypothermia affects survival is ill defined and likely varies with severity of injury. In a 1987 study, Jurkovich, Greiser, Luterman, and Curreri looked at the impact of body core hypothermia as it affected the outcome of 71 adult trauma patients with injury severity scores (ISS) greater than or equal to 25.

- 42% of patients had a core temperature below 93.2°F (34°C)
- 23% of patients had a core temperature below 91.4°F (33°C)
- 13% of patients had a core temperature below 89.6°F (32°C)

According to Jurkovich, Greiser, Luterman, and Curreri, "The mortality of hypothermia patients was consistently greater than those who remained warm, regardless of index core temperature." The authors also found that "Mortality and the incidence of hypothermia increased with higher ISS, massive fluid resuscitation, and the presence of shock. Within each subgroup (i.e., greater ISS, massive fluid administration, shock) the mortality of hypothermic patients was significantly higher than those who remained warm. No patient whose core temperature fell below 89.6°F (32°C) survived."

Hypothermia Aspect of the Lethal Triad

Hypothermia, acidosis, and coagulopathy make up the "lethal triad," a vicious cycle that leads to death in a trauma patient. Studies have shown that, by themselves, acidosis and hypothermia can impact coagulation, the body's ability to form a clot. In situations where acidosis is present in conjunction with hypothermia there is a more significant impairment of coagulation than the sum of that caused by the individual conditions. The presence of and relationship among these three conditions can result in a 90% death rate among victims of severe trauma.

Heat loss typically occurs through four different methods: radiation, conduction, convection, and evaporation (**Figure 7-1**).

Radiation is the loss or gain of heat in the form of electromagnetic energy; it is the transfer of energy from a warm object to a cooler one.

Conduction is the transfer of heat between two objects in direct contact with each other, such as a patient lying on a frozen lawn after a fall. A patient will generally lose heat faster when lying on the cold ground than when exposed to cold air. Therefore, prehospital care providers need to lift the patient off the ground in cold temperatures rather than merely covering the patient with a blanket.

Convection is the transfer of heat from a solid object to a medium that moves across that solid object, such as air or water over the body. The movement of cool air or water across the warmer skin provides for the continuous elimination of heat from the body. The body will lose heat 25 times faster in water than in air of the same temperature. A patient with wet clothing will lose body heat rapidly in mild to cold temperatures, so prehospital care providers should remove wet clothing and keep a patient dry to maintain body heat.

Evaporation of sweat from a liquid to a vapor is an extremely effective method of producing heat loss from the body, depending on the relative humidity or moisture in the air. Evaporative heat loss increases in cool, dry, and windy conditions (e.g., deserts). Collectively, convection and evaporation are more important than other methods of heat transfer because they are regulated by the body to control core temperature.

According to Moffatt ". . . spontaneous hypothermia following trauma has severely deleterious consequences for the trauma victim; however, active warming of patients can improve patient outcome. . . . Active warming of patients, to prevent spontaneous trauma-induced hypothermia, is currently the only viable method available to improve patient outcome."

Preventing Hypothermia

TECC caregivers can reduce heat loss transfer and counter hypothermia in trauma patients by taking the following actions:

- Remove wet/bloody clothing.
- Keep protective gear on or with the patient if feasible.
- Avoid cold surfaces.
- Cover casualties.
- Place blanket below patient.
- Warm intravenous (IV) fluids before administration.
- Use forced-air blanket warmers if available.

Head injury, spinal cord damage, and shock will intensify hypothermia. Consider the impact of preexisting medical conditions: thyroid disease, adrenal disease, diabetes, cardiac dysfunction, hepatic disease, autonomic nervous system dysfunction, and malnutrition.

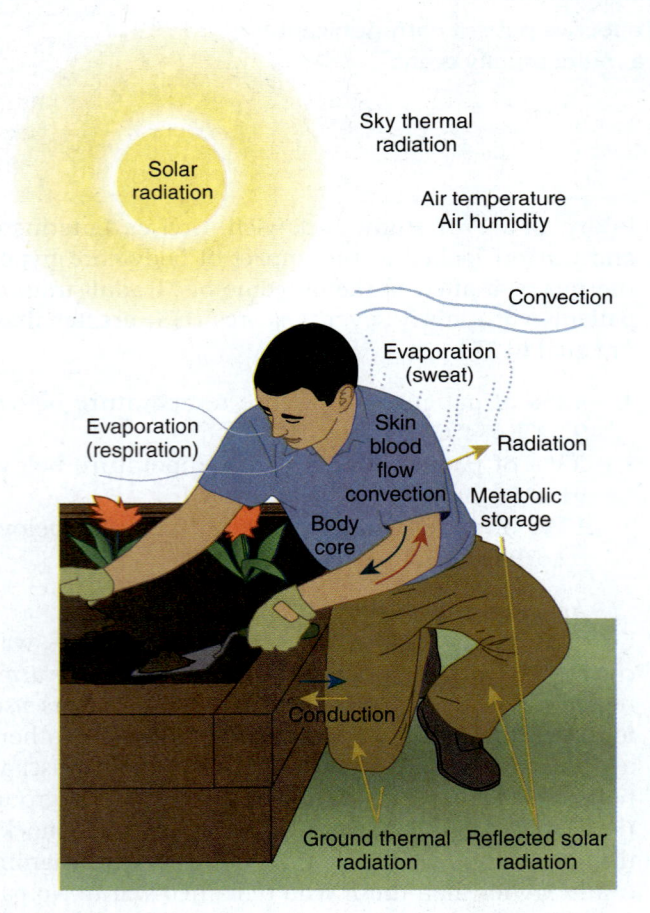

Figure 7-1 How humans exchange thermal energy with the environment.

© National Association of Emergency Medical Technicians (NAEMT).

The temperature of infused crystalloids will also impact hypothermia development. Room temperature crystalloids will reduce the patient's core temperature. If available, use warm IV solutions.

Hypothermia Prevention and Management Kits

Hypothermia prevention and management kits are recommended to prevent hypothermia. These kits have a heat-reflective shell that is wrapped around the patient. Some of the kits provide up to 10 hours of continuous dry heat with an oxygen-activated, self-heating liner that does not require an external power supply (**Figure 7-2**).

Responders must also be aware of their own potential for hypothermia and dress accordingly. Consider the three Ws when dressing in layers:

- Wicking (wool, polyester, or polypropylene)
- Warmth (down, polyester fleece, or wool)
- Wind (shell made of GORE-TEX®, or similar)

Where possible, ensure there are rewarming stations available to responders.

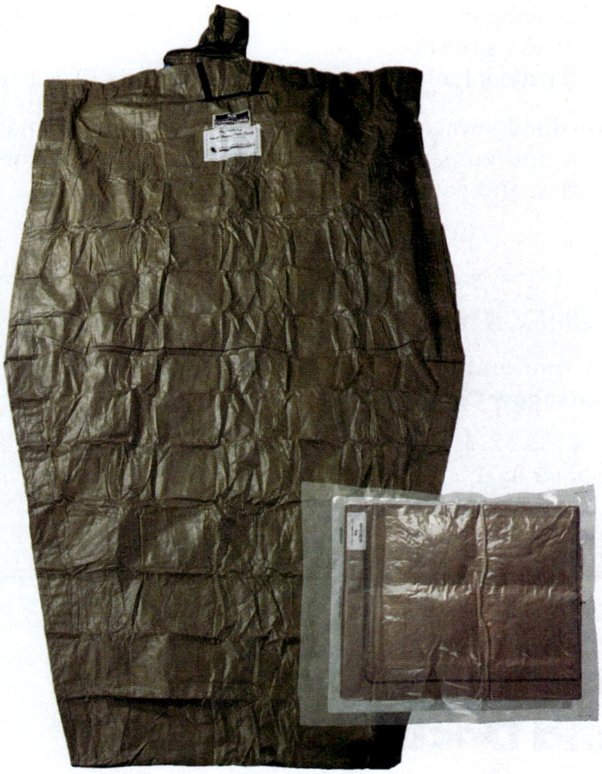

Figure 7-2 Hypothermia prevention and management kit.
Reproduced with permission from North American Rescue. Retrieved from https://www.narescue.com/nar-hypothermia-prevention-and-management-kit-hpmk

Traumatic Brain Injury Assessment and Intervention

Primary brain injury is the direct trauma to the brain and associated vascular structures that occurs at the time of the original insult. It results in contusions, hemorrhages, and lacerations and other direct mechanical injury to the brain, its vasculature, and its coverings. Because neural tissue does not regenerate well, there is minimal expectation of recovery of the structure and function lost due to primary injury. Also, little possibility exists for repair.

Glasgow Coma Scale

The Glasgow Coma Scale (GCS) is used to assess the patient's level of consciousness (**Figure 7-3**). The GCS score is calculated by using the best response noted when evaluating the patient's eyes, verbal response, and motor response. Each component of the score should be recorded individually, rather than just providing a total, so that specific changes can be noted over time. If a patient lacks spontaneous eye opening, a verbal command (e.g., "Open your eyes") should be used. If the patient does not respond to a verbal stimulus, a pressure stimulus, such as nail bed pressure with a pen or gentle squeezing of anterior axillary tissue, should be applied.

Eye Opening	Points
Spontaneous eye opening	4
Eye opening on command	3
Eye opening to pressure	2
No eye opening	1
Best Verbal Response	
Answers appropriately (oriented)	5
Gives confused answers	4
Inappropriate words	3
Makes unintelligible noises	2
Makes no verbal response	1
Best Motor Response	
Follows command	6
Localizes	5
Normal flexion response	4
Abnormal flexion response	3
Extension response	2
Gives no motor response	1
Total	

Figure 7-3 Glasgow Coma Scale.
© National Association of Emergency Medical Technicians (NAEMT).

With regard to head injury, it is generally accepted that a score of 13 to 15 likely indicates a mild traumatic brain injury (TBI), while a score of 9 to 12 is indicative of moderate TBI. A GCS score of 3 to 8 suggests severe TBI. Of course, many other factors can affect the GCS, including the presence of intoxicants or other drugs. In addition to determining the GCS, the pupils are examined quickly for symmetry and response to light. In adults, the resting pupil diameter is generally between 3 and 5 millimeters (mm). A difference of greater than 1 mm in pupil size is considered abnormal. A significant portion of the population has anisocoria, inequality of pupil size, which is either congenital or acquired as the result of ophthalmic trauma. It is not always possible in the field to distinguish between pupillary inequality caused by trauma and congenital or preexisting posttraumatic anisocoria. In the context of other evidence of significant brain injury, pupillary inequality should always be treated as secondary to the acute trauma until the appropriate workup has ruled out cerebral edema or motor or ophthalmic nerve injury.

Cushing's Triad

According to Pinto and Adeyinka, "The cranium is a rigid structure that contains three main components: brain, cerebrospinal fluid, and blood. Any increase in the volume of its contents will increase the pressure within the cranial vault." Cushing's triad is a clinical situation described by bradycardia, systolic hypertension, and irregular breathing that is caused by an increase in intracranial pressure due to a brain swelling and brain tissue hypoxia. The symptoms include the following:

- Increased systolic blood pressure, typically above 180 mm Hg
- Bradycardia
- Cheyne-Stokes respirations—slow erratic breathing, alternating with periods of apnea and rapid respirations that increase in frequency and depth and then decrease until apnea occurs again, restarting the cycle

Cushing's triad signals impending danger of brain herniation and, therefore, the need for decompression. Consider moderate hyperventilation and elevation of the head as temporizing measures. Hyperventilation will allow cerebral vessel constriction, which can lower intracranial pressure.

Intracranial Hypertension

While Cushing's triad is a clinical indication of elevated intracranial pressure, there are other symptoms that a TECC caregiver should watch for as red flags that would call for an expedited evacuation:

- Witnessed loss of consciousness
- Projectile vomiting
- Disorientation and decreased mental abilities
- Visual disturbance
- Worsening headache
- Unilateral weakness
- Abnormal speech
- Seizures

The patient may also show abnormal flexion (arms and toes toward the core) or extension (arms and toes away from body) posturing.

TBI Intervention

The key with TBI intervention is to take steps to lower the intracranial pressure while avoiding any additional injury.

- Provide enough oxygen to get to a 95% saturation, if SpO_2 monitoring is available.
- Assist with ventilations if needed: adults 10 to 12 breaths/minute, pediatric 12 to 20 breaths/minute
- Control hemorrhage.
- Insert an 18-gauge needle with a saline lock.
- If blood pressure is low, replace saline lock with an IV of lactated Ringer or normal saline. Titrate until you have a radial pulse or have a systolic blood pressure of 90 mm Hg.
- Provide spinal motion restriction if assessment indicates its need.
- If patient is not in shock, raise head at least 30 degrees.

Expedited evacuation is considered for traumatic brain-injured patients, patients with penetrating torso injuries, and patients in shock.

> **CHECK YOUR KNOWLEDGE**
>
> **A moderate traumatic brain injury would have a Glasgow Coma Scale score of:**
>
> a. 13 to 15.
> b. 9 to 12.
> c. 3 to 8.
> d. 0 to 3.

Reassess, Monitor, and Document Patient

Once all life threats have been addressed, but before you are ready to move the patient, the TECC caregiver should complete a full thorough secondary survey, apply splints, and provide monitoring in preparation of moving to the evacuation care/cold zone. However, the secondary survey should be deferred if the patient's condition is unstable in any way.

Secondary Survey

The secondary survey is a head-to-toe evaluation of a patient. The secondary survey is performed only after the primary survey is completed, all life-threatening injuries have been identified and treated, and resuscitation has been initiated. [If ongoing resuscitation is necessary, the secondary survey should be deferred or conducted during transport.] The objective of the secondary survey is to identify injuries or problems that were not identified during the primary survey. Because a well-performed primary survey will identify all life-threatening conditions, the secondary survey, by definition, deals with less serious problems. Therefore, a critical trauma patient is transported as soon as possible after conclusion of the primary survey and is not held in the field for either IV line initiation or a secondary survey.

The secondary survey uses a "look, listen, and feel" approach to evaluate the skin and everything it contains. Rather than looking at the entire body at one time, returning to listen to all areas, and, finally, returning to palpate all areas, the prehospital care provider "searches" the body. The prehospital care provider identifies injuries and correlates physical findings region by region, beginning at the head and proceeding through the neck, chest, and abdomen to the extremities, concluding with a detailed neurologic examination. The following phrases capture the essence of the entire assessment process (**Figure 7-4**):

- See, don't just look.
- Hear, don't just listen.
- Feel, don't just touch.

While examining the patient, all available information is used to formulate a patient care plan. The TECC caregiver not only provides the patient with transport but does everything possible to ensure his or her survival.

See

- Examine all of the skin of each region.
- Be attentive for external hemorrhage or signs of internal hemorrhage, such as distension of the abdomen, marked tenseness of an extremity, or an expanding hematoma.
- Note soft-tissue injuries, including abrasions, burns, contusions, hematomas, lacerations, and puncture wounds.
- Note any masses or swelling, or deformation of bones.

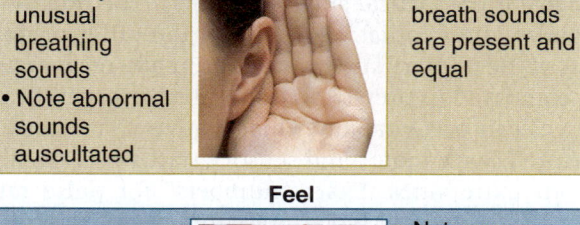

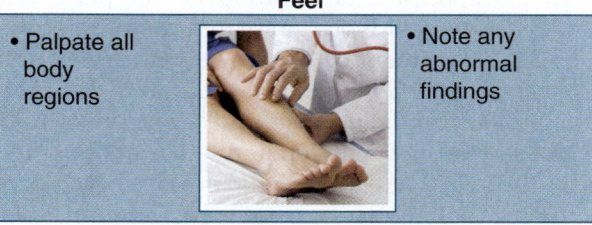

Figure 7-4 The physical assessment of a trauma patient involves careful observation, auscultation, and palpation.
© National Association of Emergency Medical Technicians (NAEMT).

See
- Be attentive for external or internal hemorrhage
- Examine all of the skin
- Note all soft tissue injuries
- Note anything that does not "look right"

Hear
- Note any unusual breathing sounds
- Note abnormal sounds auscultated
- Verify whether breath sounds are present and equal

Feel
- Palpate all body regions
- Note any abnormal findings

- Note abnormal indentations on the skin and the skin's color.
- Note anything that does not "look right."

Hear

- Note any unusual sounds when the patient inhales or exhales.
- Note any abnormal sounds when auscultating the chest.
- Check whether the breath sounds are equal in both lung fields.
- Auscultate over the carotid arteries and other vessels.
- Note any unusual sounds (bruits) over the vessels that would indicate vascular damage.

Feel

- Carefully move each bone in the region. Note any resulting crepitus, pain, or unusual movement.
- Firmly palpate all parts of the region. Note whether anything moves that should not, whether anything feels "squishy," whether the patient complains of tenderness, whether all pulses are present (and where they are felt), and whether pulsations are felt that should not be present.

During this secondary survey the TECC caregiver will inspect and dress known wounds that were previously deferred. This is also the time to consider splinting known or suspected fractures, including application of a pelvic binder if indicated.

Obtaining Vital Signs

This is the point during the indirect threat care/warm zone where the TECC provider obtains and records vital signs, if the tactical situation allows. The quality of the pulse and ventilatory rates and the other components of the primary survey are continually reevaluated and compared to previous findings because significant changes can occur rapidly. Quantitative vital signs are measured, with motor and sensory status evaluated in all four extremities. Exact "numbers" for pulse rate, ventilatory rate, and blood pressure are not critical in the initial management of the patient with severe multisystem trauma. Therefore, the measurement of the exact numbers can be delayed until completion of the essential steps of resuscitation and stabilization.

A set of complete vital signs includes blood pressure, pulse rate and quality, ventilatory rate (including breath sounds), and skin color and temperature. For the critical trauma patient, a complete set of vital signs are evaluated and recorded every 3 to 5 minutes, as often as possible, or at the time of any change in condition or a medical problem. The initial blood pressure should be taken manually. Automatic blood pressure devices may be inaccurate when the patient is significantly hypotensive; therefore, in these patients, all blood pressure measurements should be obtained manually.

Monitoring

If equipment is available, institute electronic monitoring. These include the following:

- Pulse oximetry
- Cardiac monitoring
- ETCO$_2$, if intubated
- Blood pressure

Also obtain and document vital signs using manual or electronic monitors.

Documentation

The TECC caregiver will be handing off the patient to the team in the evacuation care/cold zone area. There needs to be a transfer of information on the clinical condition of the patient, the care rendered, and any information obtained during the secondary survey. A triage tag may be the most appropriate method, particularly in the context of multiple victims (**Figure 7-5**).

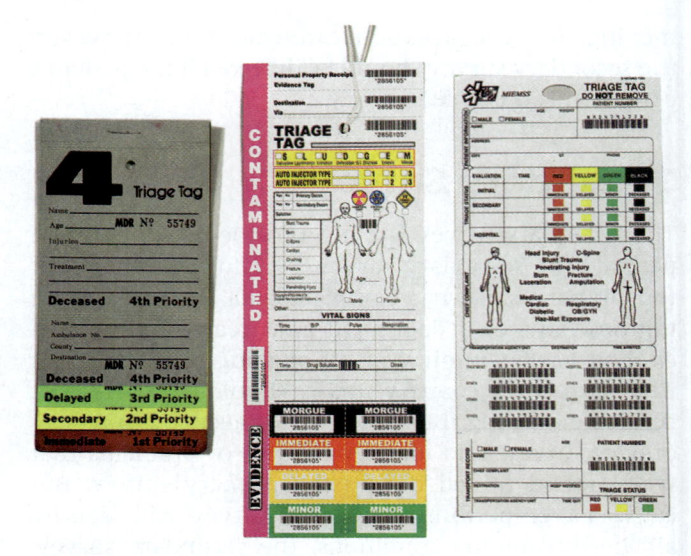

Figure 7-5 Triage tags.
© File of Life Foundation, Inc.

Communicating using triage tags can be a challenge during a dynamic mass-casualty event. During the 2017 shooting at the Route 91 Harvest country music festival in Las Vegas, casualties seeking care or transportation removed black triage tags from deceased concert-goers thinking it would get them a quicker response. Some states and agencies are experimenting with electronic tracking of patients during a mass-casualty event using radio frequency identification (RFID) triage tags. RFID tags are small electronic devices that provide data when queried with the correct radio signal. This technology can be used during mass-casualty incidents to improve the effectiveness of responders in conducting triage, treatment, transportation, and tracking of casualties to nearby hospitals.

Lacking a triage tag or form, the TECC caregiver can write on a casualty's clothing—a "Sharpie" style permanent marker is effective for this task. Under some systems the caregiver can give an oral report over a cell phone.

CHECK YOUR KNOWLEDGE

The initial blood pressure is taken:

a. on arrival to the indirect threat care/warm zone.
b. during the secondary survey.
c. just prior to leaving the indirect threat care/warm zone.
d. just prior to leaving the evacuation care/cold zone.

Analgesia

The TECC caregiver who is authorized to administer analgesics has a variety of options. For mild to moderate pain, consider oral nonnarcotic medications such as acetaminophen (Tylenol). Avoid the use of nonsteroidal anti-inflammatory drugs (NSAIDs) (e.g., aspirin, ibuprofen, naproxen, ketorolac, etc.) in the trauma patient as these medications interfere with platelet functioning and may exacerbate bleeding.

For moderate to severe pain consider the use of narcotic medications (hydrocodone, oxycodone, transmucosal fentanyl citrate, etc.) as well as ketamine at analgesic dosages. For all opiate administrations have naloxone readily available. Monitor the patient for adverse effects such as respiratory depression or hypotension. Consider adjunct administration of antiemetic medicines.

Never administer these drugs if direct and continuous monitoring of the patient is not possible afterward. Working in the dynamic indirect threat/warm zone, consider the effect of opioid-induced altered mental status on subsequent operations and required resources. It may be prudent to wait until the patient arrives at the evacuation/cold zone before administering opioids.

Ketamine

Ketamine hydrochloride is a nonopioid potent analgesic used for anesthesia. Ketamine stimulates the sympathetic nervous system and moderately increases heart rate and systolic blood pressure; these side effects might benefit trauma victims. Ketamine does not directly affect respiration or laryngeal reflexes; under ketamine analgesia and anesthesia, patients breathe spontaneously and maintain airway control. Side effects reported include dysphoria, agitation, disorientation, feeling of unreality, and nausea and vomiting.

According to Bredmose, Lockey, Grier, Watts, and Davies, ". . . the London helicopter emergency medical service has reported on their use of ketamine for analgesia and procedural sedation and concluded that ketamine is safe when used by physicians in prehospital trauma care." The military's studies show that ketamine appears to be a reliable battlefield analgesic. Ketamine's rapid onset of action and profound analgesic properties have helped it succeed where prior administration of opioids failed to provide adequate control of pain. Notably, none of the patients in their study had hallucinations or emergence phenomena, which have been associated with the anesthetic induction doses of ketamine.

> **CHECK YOUR KNOWLEDGE**
>
> **TECC choices for analgesics include all of the following, *except*:**
>
> a. acetaminophen.
> b. ketamine.
> c. aspirin.
> d. oxycodone.

Fire and Bombs as Weapons

The use of fire as a weapon dates to ancient times and remains an important element in current terrorist activities. The Mumbai terrorist attacks that occurred on November 26 to 29, 2008, demonstrated the role of fire as an element of an attack that included multiple attackers and targets, combined weapons (typically firearms and explosives), and prolonged operation to maximize media coverage (**Figure 7-6**).

The scene may include fire, intense smoke, low-to-no visibility, and the threat of firearms and explosives. Using fire as a weapon is a low-tech, low-cost tool requiring little training or technical expertise. The National Fire Protection Association (NFPA) Urban Fire Forum points out that terrorists ". . . may target locations in proximity to populated areas or large structures to maximize damage and casualties. Many residential and commercial buildings have unique characteristics that can be exploited by terrorists, including height with limited means of egress, built-in fire protection systems, and construction features that promote combustion and smoke travel."

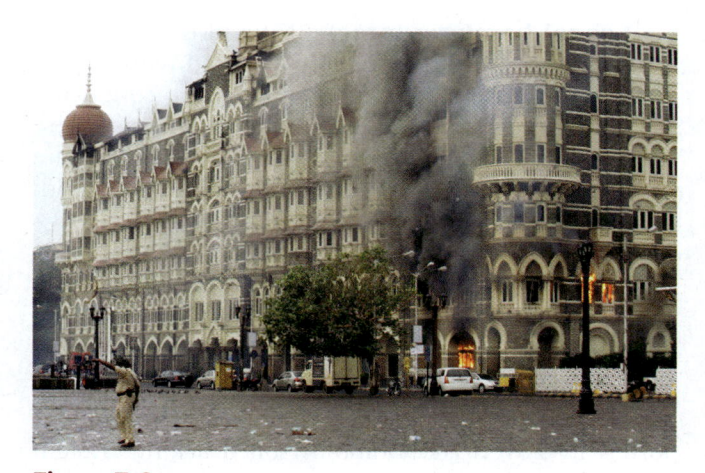

Figure 7-6 Taj Mahal Hotel set on fire by terrorists.
© Dinodia Photos/Alamy Stock Photo.

Public Safety Fire Ignition Sources

Some of the tools used by public safety can also be a source of fire at a tactical event.

- **Stun or flash bang grenade**. Remains hot for a relatively long time. Ignites combustibles where dropped. Burns flesh when picked up.
- **Explosive breaches**. A shaped charge designed to force open a door or wall. The explosion can ignite combustibles. There can be blast injuries to people that are too close to the explosive. A common injury is tympanic membrane rupture.
- **Pyrotechnic or incendiary tear gas**. A burning gas that is used for better penetration. Use by civilian special weapons and tactics (SWAT) teams; usually leads to a fire within the structure. Was used in southern California in 2013 during a deadly shoot-out with a former police officer.
- **Robotic delivery of explosives**. A technique used during the 2016 ambush and murder of five Dallas police officers. The police bomb robot was delivering a package of food to the barricaded shooter that contained an explosive device that was detonated.

Explosives

According to the annual Explosives Incident Report from the Department of Justice, there were a total of 439 bombing incidents reported in 2016, an increase of 10% from 2015; 178 of the 439 bombings targeted residential structures. Church bombings decreased from 6 to 2 incidents in 2016. Alternatively, school bombings were up by 16 incidents from 2015. The majority of the reported bombings took place at high schools and middle schools.

- **School bombing targets**. Nine of the 22 school bombings were reportedly conducted with improvised explosive devices (IEDs), 9 were conducted with explosive non-IEDs, and the remaining 4 were conducted with munitions categorized as overpressure devices. California (4), Indiana (4), and New York (3) had the highest number of incidents.
- **Residential structure targets**. Explosive non-IEDs accounted for more than half of the bombing incidents to residential structures in 2016. This is followed by IEDs at 29%, overpressure devices at 15%, and other at 5%.

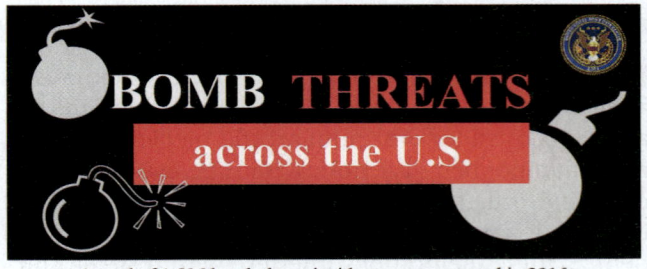

A total of 1,536 bomb threat incidents were reported in 2016. The Bomb Arson Tracking System (BATS) is the national repository for arson- and explosive-related incidents reported to the U.S. Bomb Data Center (USBDC) from law enforcement/public safety agencies (**Figure 7-7**).

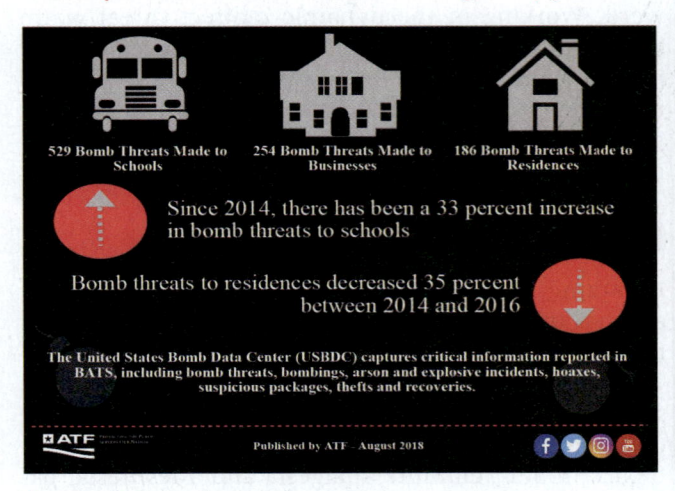

Figure 7-7 Bomb threats across the United States.
Reproduced from ATF Bomb Threats Across the United States, August 17, 2018. Retrieved from https://www.atf.gov/resource-center/infographics/bomb-threats-across-united-states

CHECK YOUR KNOWLEDGE

Which is an issue with a fire-based terror attack?

a. Intense smoke
b. Threat of explosives
c. Low-to-no visibility
d. All of these are correct.

Burn Care

Burns result from a variety of sources. While the most common etiology of burn injury is thermal, from fire or scald, other causes include chemical, electrical, and radiation exposure. Consideration of the etiology of burns will prevent the rescuer from exposing himself or herself to the burn source and sustaining unnecessary injury, as well as allow the rescuer to provide optimal care for the victim.

Large burns can be extensive, multisystem injuries capable of life-threatening effects involving the heart, lungs, kidneys, gastrointestinal tract, and immune system. The most common cause of death in a fire victim is not from the direct complications of the burn wound, but from complications of respiratory failure.

Although considered a form of trauma, burns have some significant differences from other types of trauma that merit consideration. After a trauma, such as a motor vehicle crash or a fall, the victim's physiologic response is to initiate several adaptive mechanisms to preserve life. These responses can include the shunting of blood from the periphery of the body to vital organs, increasing cardiac output, and increasing production of various protective serum proteins. In contrast, after a burn, the patient's body essentially attempts to shut down, go into shock, and die. A substantial portion of initial burn care is directed at reversal of this initial shock. In patients who have traumatic injuries as well as burns, actual mortality of these combined injuries is much greater than the combined predicted mortality of each injury individually.

Smoke inhalation is a life-threatening injury that is often more dangerous to the patient than the burn injury itself. Inhalation of toxic fumes from smoke is a greater predictor of burn mortality than the age of the patient or the size of the burn. A victim does not need to inhale a large quantity of smoke to experience a severe injury. Often, life-threatening complications from smoke inhalation may not become manifest for several days.

Assessment of Burn Injury

There are two types of measurements in assessing the burn injury: burn size estimate and burn depth. Estimation of burn size is necessary to resuscitate the patient appropriately and prevent the complications associated with hypovolemic shock from burn injury. Burn size determination is also used as a tool for stratifying injury severity and triage. The most widely applied method is the rule of nines. This method applies the principle that major regions of the body in adults are considered to be 9% of the total body surface area (TBSA).

Small burns can be assessed using the rule of palms. The use of the patient's palm has been a widely accepted and long-standing practice for estimating the size of smaller burns. The palm plus the fingers of the patient can be considered to be approximately 1% of the patient's TBSA (**Figure 7-8**).

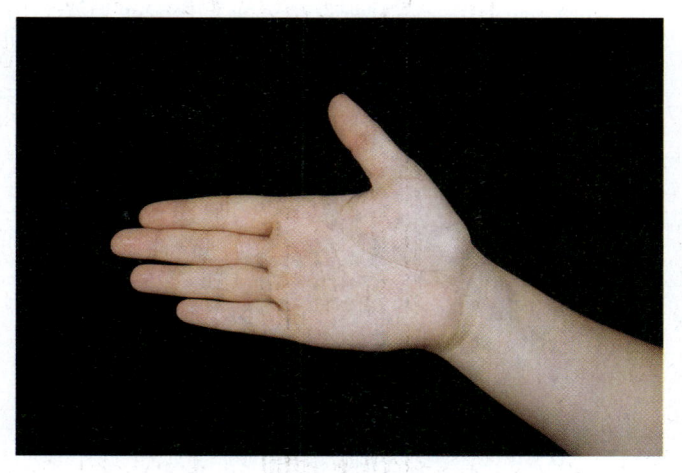

Figure 7-8 The palm method to estimate smaller burns.
© Jones & Bartlett. Photographed by Kimberly Potvin.

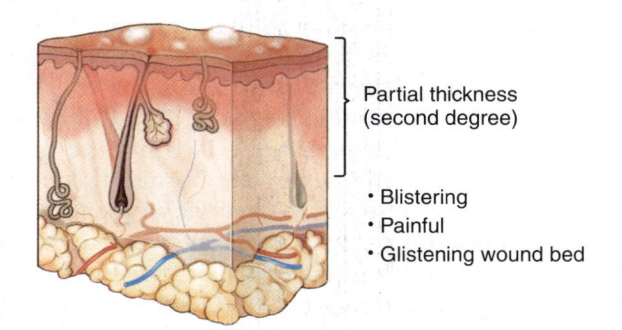

Figure 7-9 Partial-thickness burn.
© National Association of Emergency Medical Technicians (NAEMT).

Partial thickness (second degree)
- Blistering
- Painful
- Glistening wound bed

Burn depth is used to determine the severity of the injury. Partial-thickness burns, once referred to as second-degree burns, are those that involve the epidermis and varying portions of the underlying dermis. They can be further classified as either superficial or deep. Partial-thickness burns will appear as blisters or as denuded, burned areas with a glistening or wet-appearing base. These wounds are painful. Because remnants of the dermis survive, these burns can often heal in 2 to 3 weeks (**Figure 7-9**).

In partial-thickness burns, the zone of necrosis involves the entire epidermis and varying depths of the superficial dermis. If not well cared for, the zone of stasis in these injuries can progress to necrosis, making these burns larger and perhaps converting the wound to a full-thickness burn. A superficial partial-thickness burn will heal with vigilant wound care. Deep partial-thickness burns often require surgery in order to minimize scarring and prevent functional deformities of high-function areas such as the hands.

Full-thickness burns may have several appearances. Most often these wounds will appear as thick,

Figure 7-10 Full-thickness burn.
© National Association of Emergency Medical Technicians (NAEMT).

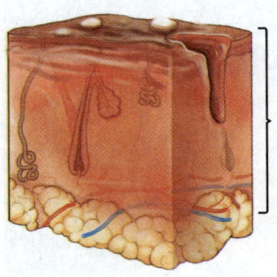

Full thickness (third degree)
- Leathery
- White to charred
- Dead tissue
- Victims will have pain from burned areas adjacent to the full-thickness burn.

dry, white, leathery burns, regardless of race or skin color. This thick leathery damaged skin is referred to as *eschar*. In severe cases, the skin will have a charred appearance with visible thrombosis (clotting) of blood vessels. Full thickness burns have, in the past, been called third-degree burns (**Figure 7-10**).

There is a common misconception that full-thickness burns are pain-free, owing to the fact that the injury destroys the nerve endings in the burned tissue. Patients with these burns may have varying degrees of pain. Full-thickness burns are typically surrounded by areas of partial-thickness and superficial burns. The nerves in these areas are intact and continue to transmit pain sensations from the damaged tissues. Burns of this depth can be disabling and life threatening. Prompt surgical excision and intensive rehabilitation at a specialized center are required.

Fluid Resuscitation of Burned Patients

Administration of large amounts of IV fluids is needed over the course of the first day postburn to prevent a patient with burns from going into hypovolemic shock. After sustaining a burn, the patient loses a substantial amount of intravascular fluid in the form of obligatory whole-body edema, as well as evaporative losses at the site of the burn. Massive fluid shifts occur, even though total body water may remain unchanged. Evaporative losses can be enormous. Excessive fluid administration, however, is harmful. Therefore, although large fluid requirements are needed to treat burn shock, too much fluid will complicate the patient's management and even worsen the patient's wounds.

The resuscitation of a patient with a burn injury is aimed not only at the restoration of the loss of intravascular volume but also at the replacement of anticipated intravascular losses at a rate that mimics those losses as they occur.

BOX 7-1

Resuscitating a Patient With a Burn Injury

Resuscitating a patient with a burn injury can be compared to filling a leaking bucket. The bucket is leaking water at a constant rate. The bucket has a line drawn inside near the top of the bucket. The objective is to keep the water level at the line. Initially the water depth will be low. The longer the bucket has been unattended, the lower the water level will be and the greater the amount of fluid that needs to be replaced. The container will continue to leak, so once the bucket has been filled to an appropriate level, water will need to be continuously added at a constant rate to maintain the desired level.

The longer the patient with a burn injury is not resuscitated or is under-resuscitated, the more hypovolemic the patient becomes. Therefore, greater amounts of fluids are required to establish a "level" of homeostasis. Once the patient has been resuscitated, the vascular space continues to leak in the same manner as the bucket. To maintain equilibrium with this homeostatic point, additional fluids need to be provided to replace the ongoing losses.

In trauma patients, the prehospital care provider is replacing the volume that the patient has already lost from hemorrhage from an open fracture or bleeding viscera. In contrast, when treating the patient with a burn injury the objective is to calculate and replace the fluids that the patient has already lost as well as replace the volume that the prehospital care provider anticipates the patient will lose over the first 24 hours after the burn injury.

The use of IV fluids, especially lactated Ringer solution, is the best way initially to manage a burn patient. Lactated Ringer is preferred to 0.9% normal saline for burn resuscitation. Burn patients typically require large volumes of IV fluids. Patients who receive large amounts of normal saline in the course of burn resuscitation can develop a condition known as hyperchloremic acidosis because of the large amounts of chloride in the normal saline solution.

Smoke Inhalation: Fluid Management Considerations

The patient with both thermal burns and smoke inhalation will require significantly more fluid than the burn patient without smoke inhalation. In an attempt to "protect the lungs," prehospital care providers will often administer less fluid than calculated. Withholding fluids increases the severity of the pulmonary injury.

Analgesia

Burns are extremely painful and, as such, require appropriate attention to pain relief beginning in the prehospital setting. Narcotic analgesics such as fentanyl (1 mg per kg body weight) or morphine (0.1 mg per kg body weight) in adequate dosages will be helpful in controlling pain.

Penetrating Eye Trauma

The increased effectiveness of combat personal protective clothing and new weapons resulted in a jump in ocular injuries, from 2.2% in World War II to 13.5% during operations in Iraq and Afghanistan. During Desert Storm soldiers encountered high-pressure spray of very fine and nearly invisible hydraulic fluids under 2,000 to 10,000 psi pressure that would blow their eyewear off when they were operating in the oil fields.

The challenge is to find appropriate eye protection that the soldiers will wear. In the United States there are 40,000 eye injuries per year. Wearing appropriate eyewear can prevent 90% of serious eye injuries.

Care for Penetrating Eye Trauma

Prehospital care is focused on protecting the eye from further trauma. Assessment of vision in the tactical arena is determining if the patient can read print, count fingers, or perceive light. TECC guidelines are different from those in traditional emergency medical services (EMS) textbooks and recommend the use of a rigid eye shield without padding. The objective is to provide a hard barrier between the impaled eye and the environment. Any padding under the rigid shield may stick to the eye or increase intraocular pressure. Increased intraocular pressure could result in loss of vitreous fluid from an injured eye.

In a tactical situation, it is preferred to leave the uninjured eye uncovered, so the casualty can move and respond to changes in the indirect threat/warm zone conditions. If both eyes have to be covered, assure that a TECC caregiver is providing verbal support and direction.

If the patient's vision is decreasing and the area around the eye is rapidly swelling, this is an urgent situation. There may be a hemorrhage behind the eye that is endangering the integrity of the eyeball.

> **CHECK YOUR KNOWLEDGE**
>
> A secondary survey reveals a small piece of shrapnel imbedded in the patient's eye. TECC guidelines call for the caregiver to:
>
> a. initiate a 20-minute flush with saline solution.
> b. prepare and place a doughnut ring around the shrapnel.
> c. tape a rigid eye shield over the injured eye.
> d. cover both eyes with occlusive dressing.

Moving and Communicating With the Patient

The goal is to get the casualty out of the indirect threat care/warm zone and into the evacuation care/cold zone. This requires coordination with the incident management team and the security status of the hot zone threats.

Since the indirect threat care/warm zone is probably an austere environment, some creativity may be required to move casualties who are unable to walk. TECC caregivers may need to improvise stretchers or utilize lift techniques (**Figure 7-11**).

The path from the indirect threat care/warm zone to the evacuation care/cold zone may have changed, and the TECC caregivers may be required to create a new path by breaching a wall or moving in a different direction to maintain a safe passageway.

Communicating With the Patient

In preparing for the move, reassure the casualty that the situation is improving and direct the person to

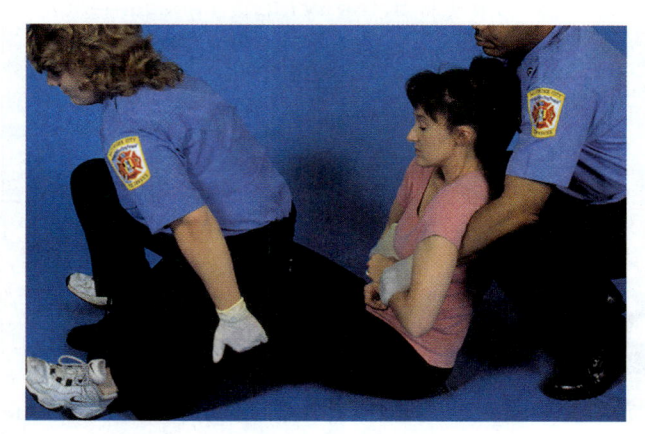

Figure 7-11 Extremity lift.

continue self-care. This event creates high anxiety and emotions, with casualties and caregivers hypervigilant. In some situations, the casualty may be a TECC responder.

Your role is to be calm, clear, and consistent in message, instructions, and demeanor. There will be challenges with parents of injured children and colleagues of injured responders. Each wants the best for the victim, and this may require tact and a command presence from you as the caregiver. Some caregivers have had success when assigning tasks to the "worried well" that would be appropriate based on the current situation.

Communicating With Receiving Hospitals

By the time casualties are moving out of the indirect threat/warm zone, local hospitals have mobilized their teams to receive patients. Whether directly or through the medical sector in the incident management system, provide hospitals with the number of patients, conditions, and prehospital treatment.

Based on experience with recent incidents, nearby hospitals may already be busy with casualties that bypassed EMS and went directly to the hospital. The goal of the transportation sector in the incident management system is to get each casualty to the most appropriate hospital.

> **CHECK YOUR KNOWLEDGE**
>
> **When preparing to move casualties from the indirect threat care/warm zone to the evacuation care/cold zone:**
>
> a. wait for the appropriate number of ambulance teams to arrive at the warm zone/cold zone border.
> b. coordinate with the incident management team.
> c. determine the smoothest path with the fewest obstacles.
> d. take the same path you used to get to the indirect threat care/warm zone.

CPR in a Multicasualty Event

Traumatic cardiac arrest (TCA) represents a unique problem and poses difficult challenges in the care of trauma patients. The literature has suggested that attempted resuscitation from TCA in trauma is futile and consumptive of medical and human resources.

Recent research indicates some success in resuscitation of TCA patients delivered to the emergency department despite not achieving restoration of spontaneous circulation (ROSC) during prehospital care.

Working in the austere environment of multiple patients in a tactical situation places the TECC caregivers in a dilemma. Do they focus all of their resources on one patient, or do they try to make a difference to as many patients as their resources and time allow?

Correct Tension Pneumothorax

Based on the military's experience, the TECC guidelines have the caregiver consider bilateral needle decompression for nonbreathing and pulseless casualties with torso or polytrauma (two or more significant trauma injuries). This is to rule out tension pneumothorax as the cause of the cardiac arrest before discontinuing care. In one study, 4 of the 18 TCA patients receiving chest decompressions had a return of cardiac output.

> **CHECK YOUR KNOWLEDGE**
>
> **While triaging patients in the indirect threat care/warm zone you encounter a casualty with multiple system trauma who has no pulse. The TECC recommendation is to:**
>
> a. triage patient as gray or black tag.
> b. perform the head tilt maneuver to see if respiration returns.
> c. do three cycles of continuous closed chest compressions, and then check for a pulse.
> d. perform bilateral needle chest decompressions, and then check for a pulse.

Summary

- Prevent hypothermia.
- Effectively manage TBI.
- Administer pain management following local protocols.
- Provide burn care; stop the burning process.
- Use a shield for penetrating eye injuries.
- CPR is not warranted in multipatient incidents (there are few exceptions). Consider bilateral needle chest decompressions if evidence of thoracic trauma is present.

REFERENCES AND RESOURCES

Ari AB. Eye injuries on the battlefields of Iraq and Afghanistan: public health implications. *Optometry.* 2006;77:329-339.

Blanch RJ, Scott RAH. Military ocular injury: presentation, assessment and management. *J R Army Med Corps.* 2009;155(4):279-284.

Bredmose PP, Lockey DJ, Grier G, Watts B, Davies G. Pre-hospital use of ketamine for analgesia and procedural sedation. *Emerg Med J.* 2009;26(1):62-64.

Chinn M, Colella MR. An evidence-based review of prehospital traumatic cardiac arrest. *J Emerg Med Serv.* 2017 Apr;42(4):26-32.

Häske D, Böttiger BW, Bouillon B, et al. Analgesia in patients with trauma in emergency medicine. *Deutsches Arzteblatt Int.* 2017;114(46):785-792.

Jurkovich GJ, Greiser WB, Luterman A, Curreri PW. Hypothermia in trauma victims: an ominous predictor of survival. *J Trauma.* 1987;27(9):1019-1024.

Konesky KL, Guo WA. Revisiting traumatic cardiac arrest: should CPR be initiated? *Eur J Trauma Emer Surg.* 2018;44(6):903-908.

Losvik OK, Murad MK, Skjerve E, Husum H. Ketamine for prehospital trauma analgesia in a low-resource rural trauma system: a retrospective comparative study of ketamine and opioid analgesia in a ten-year cohort in Iraq. *Scand J Trauma Resus Emerg Med.* 2015;23(1):94.

Lyon R, Schwan C, Zeal J, et al. Successful use of ketamine as a prehospital analgesic by pararescuemen during Operation Enduring Freedom: our experience and literature review. *J Spec Oper Med.* 2018;18(1):69-73.

Miatry N, Bleetman A, Roberts KJ. Chest decompression during the resuscitation of patients in prehospital traumatic cardiac arrest. *Emerg Med J.* 2009;26(10):738-740.

Moffatt SE. Hypothermia in trauma. *Emerg Med J.* 2013;30:989-996.

National Association of Emergency Medical Technicians. *PHTLS: Prehospital Trauma Life Support.* 9th ed. Burlington, MA: Public Safety Group; 2019.

National Association of EMS Physicians, American College of Surgeons. Withholding of resuscitation for adult traumatic cardiopulmonary arrest. *Prehosp Emerg Care.* 2013;17(2):291.

Perlman R, Callum J, Laflamme C, et al. A recommended early goal-directed management guideline for the prevention of hypothermia-related transfusion, morbidity, and mortality in severely injured trauma patients. *Crit Care (London, England).* 2016;20(1):107.

Pfeifer JW. Fire as a weapon in terrorist attacks. *CTC Sentinel.* 2013;6(7):5-8.

Pinto VL, Adeyinka A. Increased intracranial pressure. [Updated 2019 Jan 20]. *StatPearls.* https://www.ncbi.nlm.nih.gov/books/NBK482119/. Accessed February 20, 2019.

Urban Fire Forum. *UFF Position Statement: Fire and Smoke as a Weapon.* Quincy, MA: National Fire Protection Association; 2014.

LESSON 8

Evacuation Care/Cold Zone

LESSON OBJECTIVES
- Describe the differences between indirect threat care/warm zone and evacuation care/cold zone.
- Explore the multiple transport platforms available in a tactical event.
- Understand the need to transport the right patient, to the right place, at the right time.
- Describe the additional medical resources available for use in evacuation care/cold zone.

Overview of Evacuation Care/Cold Zone

Lesson 8: Evacuation Care/Cold Zone gets the casualty moved from indirect threat care/warm zone to evacuation care/cold zone.

Differences Between Indirect Threat Care/Warm Zone and Evacuation Care/Cold Zone

The cold zone is an area where it is relatively safe to provide care. For a vast majority of civilian emergencies, this is the where emergency medical services (EMS) care is delivered prior to moving to a transport vehicle. For tactical emergency casualty care (TECC) providers this is evacuation care—the kind of casualty care provided by TECC caregivers after rescuing casualties from a dangerous place.

Most of the MARCH casualty care techniques detailed in the indirect threat/warm zone came with the caution that the care was dependent upon the current threat situation. The dynamic and fluid nature of threats may have resulted in the casualty care technique being deferred until the casualty was in the evacuation/cold zone. The indirect threat/warm zone is an area where the threat is intermediate between the hot and cold zones; this is often the most challenging zone regarding medical decision making. The benefit of a particular intervention must be considered relative to the risk of additional injury to the casualty or the caregiver. Certain actions considered standard for care in normal situations, such as applying a cervical collar for penetrating neck injuries before moving the casualty, make no sense in a tactical environment. Some casualty-critical techniques that were started in the hot or warm zone must now be reassessed and completed in the cold zone.

Situational Awareness in Evacuation Care/Cold Zone

TECC caregivers and incident managers must maintain vigilance even in the evacuation/cold zone.

- Responders may be a target as they respond into and out of the evacuation/cold zone.
- Secondary devices may be placed at the predesignated staging and loading areas.
- There may be direct attacks along routes of travel.
- The direct threat may move into the evacuation/cold zone.
- Casualties being moved to the evacuation/cold zone may be part of the attacking force and reengage during transport or upon arrival at the evacuation/cold zone.
- Ambulance vehicles have been used as decoys, weapons caches, or bombs in international events.

Two trends reinforce the need for continuing active situational awareness while operating in the evacuation/cold zone: (1) Lone wolf actors, and (2) a trend toward harming first responders. Maggie Koerth-Baker, reporting for FiveThirtyEight.com, shared this observation: "Lone-wolf terrorists are also the more deadly terrorists, according to a 2017 study published in the journal *Terrorism and Political Violence*. That's largely because we have strong counterterrorism law enforcement operations that make it difficult for group terrorism to operate effectively. Lone wolves tend to be more educated and more socially isolated than other kinds of terrorists." As of 2015, lone wolf actors accounted for 6% of terrorists in the United States, but they were responsible for 25% of attacks.

EMS and fire responders have become targets. They have been purposefully ambushed upon arrival at an emergency incident, where they found themselves immediately under hostile gunfire. A 2012 structure fire on Christmas Eve morning in rural New York resulted in all four members of the first-arriving engine company getting shot, two fatally. A predawn 2018 structure fire and ambush in Oregon included shotgun blasts into the engine as they arrived at the burning house.

In Ferguson, Missouri, civil unrest started rapidly after a white police officer shot a black suspect in August 2014. From the start, public safety was hampered by constant gunfire, especially in the evening/overnight period. Shells left by the protestors included semiautomatic arms like the AR-15. This required fire fighters to leave active-fire scenes. EMS crews operating in cold zones suddenly found themselves in a hot zone as the crowds surged.

Have Primary, Secondary, and Tertiary Evacuation Plans

The dynamic nature of tactical events requires TECC caregivers to balance medical care with operational risk assessments. The PACE methodology helps with evacuation planning:

- Primary: Transportation of casualties from evacuation zone using ambulances and medical helicopters
- Alternate: Transportation of casualties using alternate emergency service vehicles, such as an ambulance bus or SUV
- Contingency: Nontraditional transport vehicles such as armored or commercial vehicles as well as boats or rail transport
- Emergency: Ad hoc methods based on resources available and immediate casualty and security conditions

In addition to the mode of casualty movement, the route to get from the evacuation/cold zone to a medical facility may be impacted by weather, blocked roads, or a direct threat that has moved. TECC caregivers also need to apply PACE to the routes to medical facilities.

Evacuation Care Transport Resources

The preferred transport method is to use conventional EMS transport resources. That means fully stocked ambulances with appropriately credentialed caregivers, either paramedic or EMT. At this point, casualty care is no longer dependent on what TECC caregivers carried to the casualties.

Local EMS providers know their service area and the capabilities of the receiving medical facilities, and they will be operating under an incident management system that usually includes regional coordination of casualty destination. Many urban regions also have ambulance buses that can transport up to a dozen casualties (**Figure 8-1**).

Air medical transport can move critically injured casualties rapidly to trauma, burn, or specialty centers. It has a wider transport range that will allow the critical casualties to be moved to more distant hospitals to reduce the impact on the closest specialty centers. Air medical caregivers tend to have a higher level of training and more advanced equipment than the local ambulance-based service. Availability of rotary wing vehicles is often impacted by weather and flight rules.

TECC caregivers may need to consider unconventional transport vehicles. Law enforcement patrol vehicles and EMS utility vehicles can be used to transport casualties. Armored vehicles can hold two to three casualties.

Civilian buses and commercial trucks can transport multiple stable casualties, often with a single EMS provider supplying oversight and driving directions. Do not rule out boats or rail transportation, based on the geography and status of the evacuation routes.

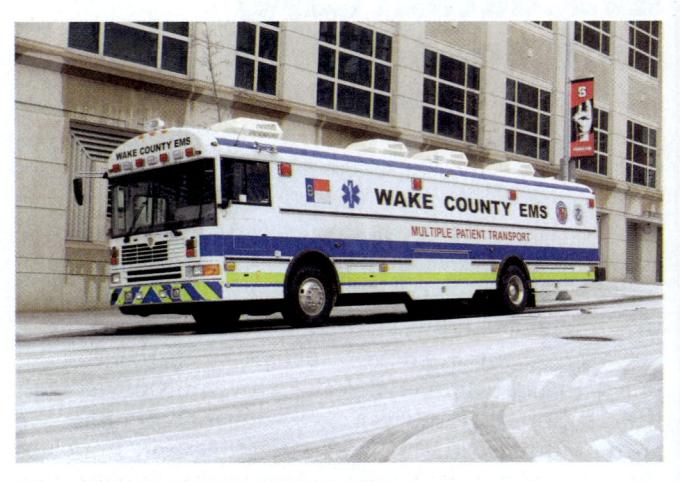

Figure 8-1 Ambulance bus.
© Mike Legeros. Used with permission.

> **CHECK YOUR KNOWLEDGE**
>
> **Evacuation care means medical care:**
>
> a. delivered upon arrival to a hospital or medical center.
> b. provided during transport from the cold zone to the hospital or medical center.
> c. provided while the casualty is in the cold zone.
> d. provided during the movement of the casualty from the warm zone to the cold zone.

Evacuation Care: Reassessment

There are two significant changes when the casualty arrives at the evacuation care/cold zone. There are more caregivers and resources available, and there is an immediate need to reassess the casualty's condition and the effectiveness of the care provided in the warm zone. While the element creating the hot zone threat may still be uncontrolled, the evacuation/cold zone allows a more comprehensive casualty medical evaluation with a more robust delivery of care.

> **CHECK YOUR KNOWLEDGE**
>
> **A significant difference in evacuation care/cold zone is:**
>
> a. better ventilation and lighting.
> b. more caregivers and resources available.
> c. ability to interact with the incident commander.
> d. tighter security.

Airway

Confirm existing airway device, if used, is in the proper place. Determine if spinal motion restrictions are required, if not already implemented. Administer oxygen if available. The evacuation care/cold zone may be the first time oxygen is available.

If the airway is patent, continue with reassessment. If not, replace with supraglottic device or endotracheal intubation as appropriate based on the overall patient condition.

Supraglottic Airways

Supraglottic airways offer a functional alternative to endotracheal intubation. Many jurisdictions allow use of these devices because minimal training is required to achieve and retain competency. These devices are inserted without direct visualization of the vocal cords. The primary advantage of supraglottic airways is that they may be inserted independent of the patient's position, which may be especially important in trauma patients with access and extrication difficulties or a high suspicion of cervical injury.

When placed into a patient, supraglottic airways are designed to isolate the trachea from the esophagus. None of these devices provides a complete seal of the trachea; therefore, while the risk of aspiration is lowered, it is not completely eliminated. Some manufacturers have developed supraglottic airways in pediatric sizes. TECC caregivers should ensure proper sizing according to the manufacturer's specifications if using these types of airways on pediatric patients (**Figure 8-2**).

Indications

- Basic providers. If the prehospital care provider is trained and authorized and cannot easily ventilate the apneic or bradypneic patient with a bag-mask device and an OPA or NPA, a supraglottic airway is the primary airway device.
- Advanced providers. A supraglottic airway is often the alternative airway device when the prehospital care provider is unable to perform endotracheal intubation and cannot easily ventilate the patient with a bag-mask device and an oropharyngeal or nasopharyngeal airway.

Contraindications

- Provider is able to adequately ventilate the patient with a bag-mask device and an OPA or NPA
- Intact gag reflex

Complications

- Gagging and vomiting, if gag reflex is intact
- Aspiration
- Damage to the esophagus
- Hypoxia if ventilated using the incorrect lumen

> **CHECK YOUR KNOWLEDGE**
>
> **The primary advantage of using a supraglottic airway is that it:**
>
> a. provides positive control of the trachea.
> b. completely eliminates the risk of aspiration.
> c. introduces high concentrations of oxygen.
> d. may be inserted independent of the patient's position.

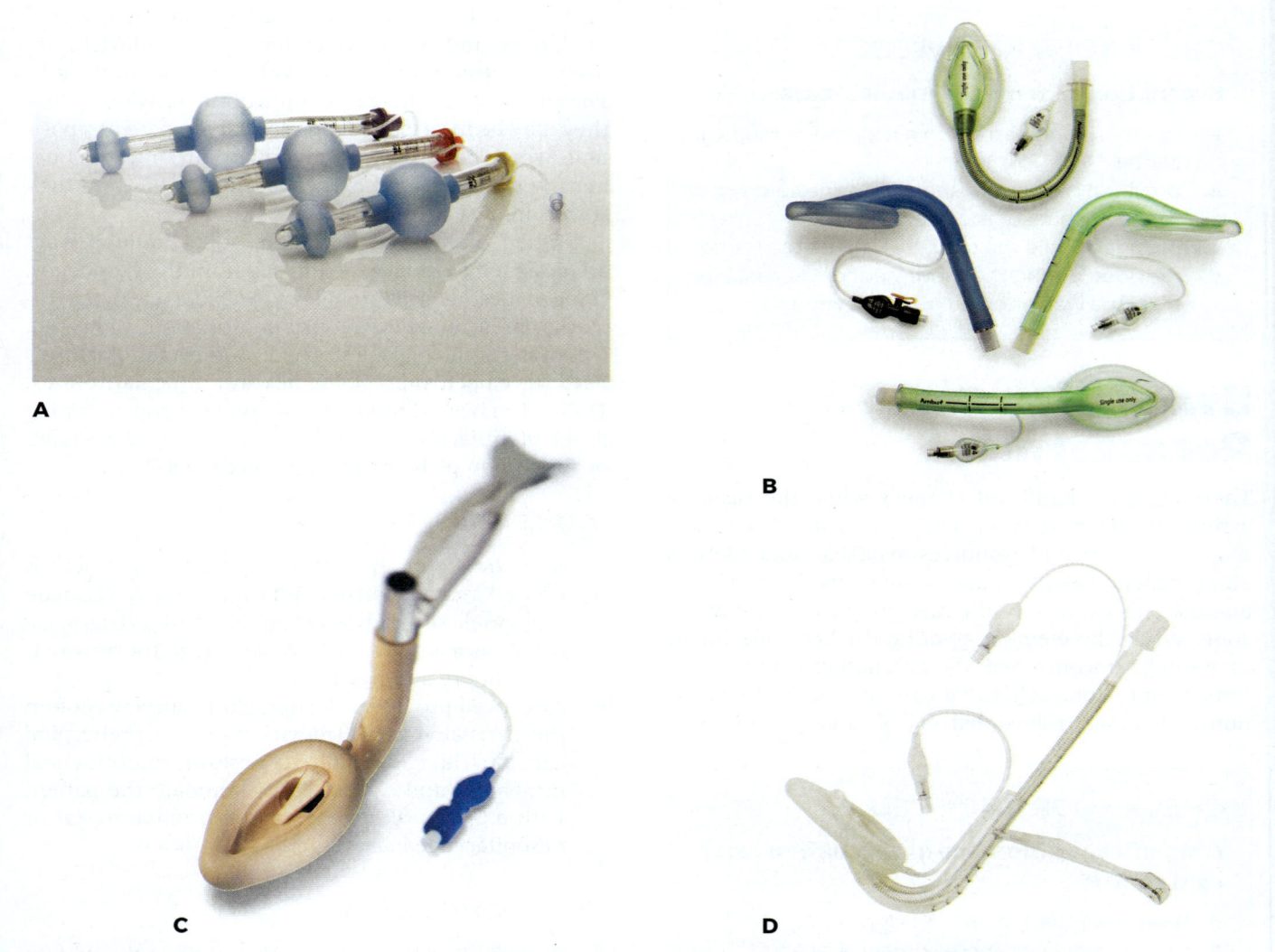

Figure 8-2 **A.** King laryngotracheal airway. **B.** Laryngeal mask airway (LMA). **C.** Intubating LMA. **D.** Intubating LMA with endotracheal tube in place.
Source: Courtesy of Ambu, Inc. (**A–B**), and Courtesy of Teleflex, Inc. (**C, D**).

Breathing

Observe that existing chest seals are working appropriately and the patient is not developing a tension pneumothorax. Treat all open pneumothoraces with a vented or nonvented occlusive chest seal. Look for hypoxia or respiration-related hypotension. Burp existing chest seal. If the clinical condition remains the same or worsens, perform a needle decompression. Management of a tension pneumothorax is no different in the evacuation care/cold zone than it was in the indirect threat/warm zone.

Needle Decompression

For needle decompression, the preferred approach is through the fourth or fifth intercostal space along the anterior axillary line (**Figure 8-3**). It can also be performed through the second or third intercostal space in the midclavicular line of the involved side of the chest.

During needle decompression, the needle and catheter should be advanced until the return of a rush of air is achieved and advanced no farther (**Figure 8-4**). Once decompression is achieved, the catheter is taped to the chest to prevent dislodgement (**Figure 8-5**). Improper placement (location or depth) may result in injuries to the lungs, heart, or great vessels.

As a general rule, a bilateral tension pneumothorax is exceedingly rare in patients who are not intubated and ventilated with positive pressure. The first step in reassessing the patient is to confirm the location of the endotracheal tube, ensure that it has no kinks or bends causing compression of the tube, and ensure that the tube has not inadvertently moved down into

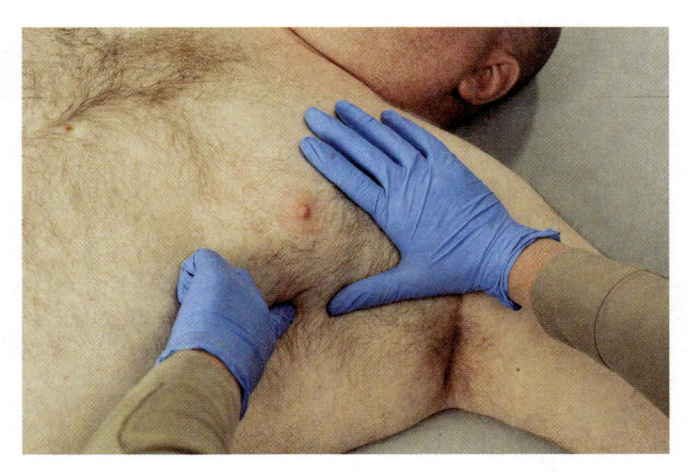

Figure 8-3 Needle decompression of the thoracic cavity is most easily accomplished and produces the least chance for complication if it is done at the fifth intercostal space at the anterior axillary line.
© Jones & Bartlett Learning.

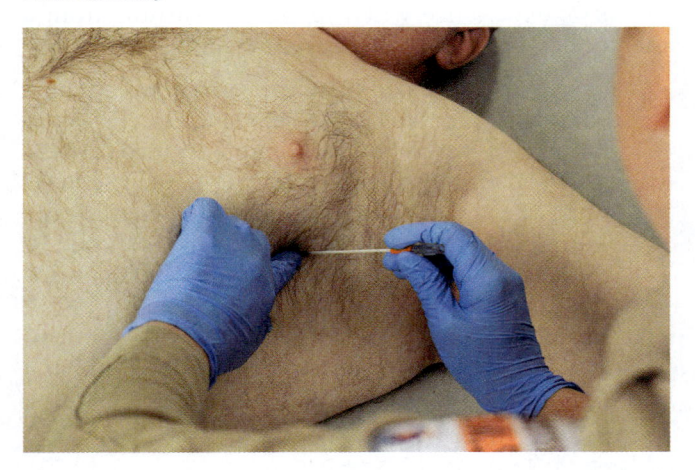

Figure 8-4 The needle and catheter should be advanced until the return of a rush of air is achieved and advanced no farther.
© Jones & Bartlett Learning. Photographed by Darren Stahlman.

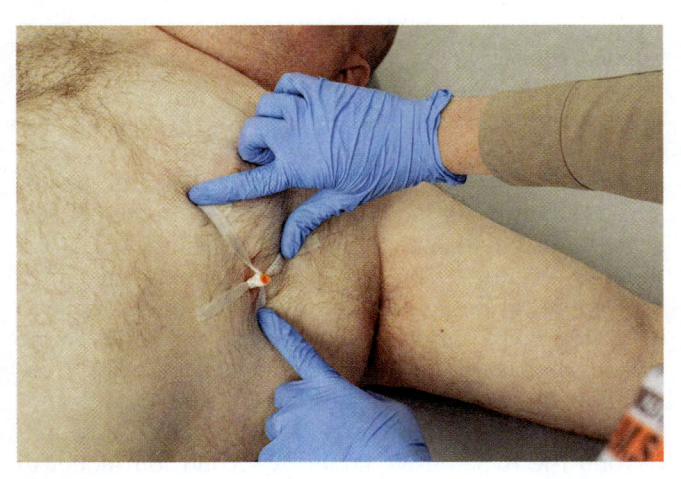

Figure 8-5 Once decompression is achieved, the catheter is taped to the chest to prevent dislodgement.
© Jones & Bartlett Learning.

a main bronchus. Extreme caution should be exercised with bilateral needle decompression in patients who are not being ventilated with positive-pressure ventilation. If the prehospital care provider's assessment is in error, the creation of bilateral pneumothoraces can cause severe respiratory distress.

The patient should be rapidly transported to an appropriate facility. IV access should be obtained unless transport time is particularly short. The patient must be closely observed for deterioration. Repeat decompression and endotracheal intubation may become necessary.

> **CHECK YOUR KNOWLEDGE**
>
> A needle decompression requires an IV needle of _____ gauge or larger.
>
> a. 22
> b. 20
> c. 18
> d. 16

Evacuation Care: Hemorrhage Control

Observe the casualty for signs of active bleeding. Confirm that there is an absence of distal pulses in extremities where a tourniquet has been applied. Observe hemostatic dressings for additional bleeding.

Perform a complete blood sweep. Blood sweeps only work well with clean gloves, major hemorrhage, and light. A combination of raking and sweeping is more effective. *Raking* means you assess by spreading your fingers out and curving them in, resembling a rake you would you use to remove leaves from a lawn. Your fingers will detect wounds that may be missed under bloody clothes. Expose and access each wound found.

A blood sweep-and-rake assessment is similar to the emergency medical technician/paramedic physical head-to-toe secondary assessment. This is a much more detailed assessment than the sweep done in the indirect threat/warm zone. When performing the blood sweep-and-rake procedure, your hands rapidly palpate from head to toe and search for any hemorrhaging wounds that were not identified after the visual size-up.

Tranexamic Acid

Tranexamic acid (TXA) reduces blood loss by inhibiting the enzymatic breakdown of fibrin. The CRASH-2 trial has shown that administration of TXA to bleeding trauma patients who are within 3 hours of injury significantly reduces death due to bleeding and all-cause mortality, without increasing the risk of vascular occlusive events. TXA is a synthetic derivative of lysine that inhibits fibrinolysis by blocking the lysine binding sites on plasminogen.

Use of TXA in the prehospital setting is controversial, and safety and efficacy have not been established. That said, many services are beginning to use it. If your service is using TXA in the out-of-hospital environment, these are the indications and the techniques for its use. TXA should be administered as soon as possible for patients with the potential for significant blood transfusions due to multiple amputations, severe uncontrolled internal bleeding, or hemorrhagic shock. In the tactical scene, the evacuation/cold zone may be the first opportunity for TXA administration. Do not administer TXA if the injury is more than 3 hours old.

TXA is administered as 1 gram via IV or IO access under a slow, 10-minute infusion. Be aware of transient hypotension during administration. Onset of action is within 5 to 15 minutes of application. The duration of fibrinolysis clot blocking is 3 hours.

TXA can also be administered orally or directly on the bleeding site. Contraindications include severe renal insufficiency and hematuria (blood in urine). Complications include nausea, vomiting, and diarrhea; allergy; and occasional orthostatic tendency (transient hypotension). There is a theoretical risk of deep vein thrombosis.

> **CHECK YOUR KNOWLEDGE**
>
> **Assessing the casualty for hemorrhage includes:**
>
> a. loosening tourniquets applied in the hot zone.
> b. performing the rake procedure.
> c. palpating systolic blood pressure.
> d. blanching fingernails.

Tourniquet Assessment and Conversion

During your blood sweep, reassess the effectiveness and clinical indications of tourniquets that were applied in the hot or cold zone. Is the wound appropriate for tourniquet use? If not, use a pressure dressing or other technique to control the bleeding. However, do not consider tourniquet removal unless severely prolonged transport time is anticipated.

Is the hemorrhage controlled? Are there no distal pulses below the tourniquet? If the hemorrhage is not controlled or distal pulses are present, tighten the existing tourniquet or apply an additional tourniquet. Tourniquets can remain in place if the time to travel from evacuation/cold zone care to a receiving medical facility is not substantially more than 2 hours.

Tourniquet conversion is the process of exchanging an applied tourniquet for a hemostatic agent or a pressure dressing. While an effective tool in the hot or warm zones, the extended application of a tourniquet for substantially more than 2 hours during evacuation and transportation to definitive medical care may create avoidable damage—damage such as pressure injury to the tissue compressed or ischemic injury to the tissue not getting blood flow.

Tourniquet Conversion Procedures

Guidelines for tourniquet conversion are based on the military's experience when removing warriors from a theater of war to a forward surgical team.

- Tourniquet conversion should be considered each time the casualty is moved to the next level of care (hot to warm, warm to cold, cold to community medical facility, or community medical facility to trauma center).
- While the upper limit has not been scientifically determined, field tourniquet conversions should be considered for up to 6 hours after the initial tourniquet application.
- Tourniquet conversion of a casualty with a tourniquet applied for over 6 hours should be done in a community hospital or trauma center.

Plus-1 Tourniquet

The military's approach to tourniquet management includes a "Plus-1" tourniquet. Add one loose tourniquet to each extremity to which a tourniquet has already been applied (Plus 1). This is done for two reasons. The first reason is that if the tourniquet that is already in place breaks during the conversion process, there is already a backup in place ready to be tightened. Tourniquets are subject to environmental degradation and significant wear and tear during application. In an after-action report distributed with the 2014 Committee on TCCC meeting minutes, 10% of the tourniquets used in a six-patient casualty incident broke while being applied.

The second reason is that it is difficult to determine where the patient is on the resuscitation curve. Administration of fluids (crystalloids, colloids, or blood) and/or ketamine has the potential to raise blood pressure beyond the hypotensive target. A second tourniquet in place reduces bleeding time if bleeding suddenly reoccurs (**Figure 8-6**).

With the Plus-1 tourniquet in place, loosen the first tourniquet. If no bleeding from the wound is noted, then

LESSON 8 Evacuation Care/Cold Zone 89

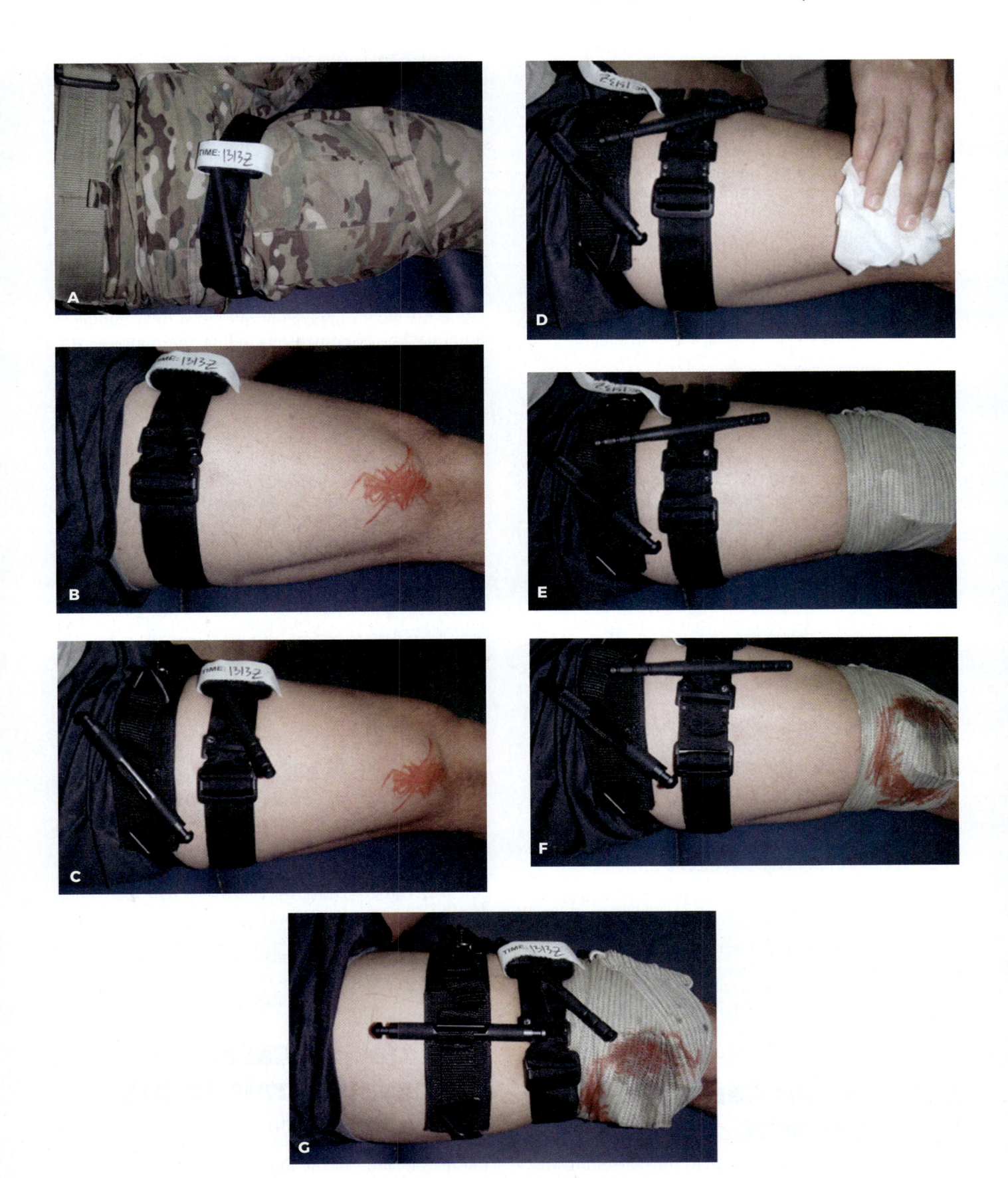

Figure 8-6 A second tourniquet in place reduces bleeding time if bleeding suddenly reoccurs.

Brendon Drew, DO; David Bird, PA-C, MPAS; Michael Matteucci, MD; Sean Keenan, MD, Tourniquet Conversion A Recommended Approach in the Prolonged Field Care Setting, *Journal of Special Operations Medicine* Volume 15, Edition 3/Fall 2015.

leave both tourniquets in place but not tightened and dress the wound. If bleeding is noted, apply a hemostatic agent and hold pressure for 3 to 5 minutes. If no further bleeding is noted, leave both loose tourniquets in place and dress the wound. If hemostatic agents fail to control the bleeding, tighten the original tourniquet in as distal a position as possible to control the bleeding. Ensure the distal pulse is absent. Leave the Plus-1 tourniquet loose and proximal to the tightened tourniquet.

Contraindications for Tourniquet Conversion

When should tourniquets not be converted? There should be no attempt to convert tourniquets used for amputations. The tourniquet should be placed high and tight on the extremity—near the axilla for upper extremity amputations and near the groin for the lower extremity. Another contraindication to tourniquet conversion is the inability to monitor the patient directly. The inability to observe the casualty in the event of rebleeding is a contraindication to conversion. This includes patients wrapped in blankets or other hypothermia-prevention materials. Conversion should not be attempted if the extremity cannot be observed for active rebleeding.

Conversion should not be attempted on a patient in shock. If there is any concern for hemorrhagic shock, resuscitation must be initiated prior to attempted tourniquet conversion. A tourniquet should never be periodically loosened to give the tissue oxygen and blood. This results in "incremental exsanguination." In other words, the patient is bled to death in short bursts. A tourniquet should only be loosened during conversion.

Most importantly, tourniquet conversion should never be considered unless time from initial application to arrival at the emergency department will substantially exceed 2 hours.

> **CHECK YOUR KNOWLEDGE**
>
> **Which is a contraindication for tourniquet conversion?**
>
> a. Utilization of the pelvic binder
> b. Lack of hemostatic agent
> c. Patient has received colloids or whole blood.
> d. Transport time to the hospital is anticipated to be 90 minutes.

Evacuation Care: Shock Management

The pleural space, abdominal cavity, mediastinum, and retroperitoneum are all spaces that can hold enough blood to cause death from exsanguination. The body's response to shock changes as blood loss continues. The body increases the heart rate and constricts the blood vessels to maintain organ perfusion during compensated shock. This presents as a patient with a normal blood pressure reading and possibly a rapid thready pulse. Casualties may be agitated, restless, or anxious.

Continued blood loss results in decompensated shock. The pulse and respiration rates continue to rise as the blood pressure starts to fall. The patient will become lethargic. The skin will look pale or ashen, with a clammy feel. Near the end-stage the pulse rate will fall as the blood supply continues to shrink. Complete a full patient assessment, including vital signs, as you would a trauma patient outside of a tactical area.

Establish IV or Intraosseous (IO) Line

While in the indirect threat/warm zone, an 18-gauge needle with a saline lock is the recommended vascular access. Now that the casualty is in the evacuation/cold zone, more appropriate shock management procedures can be used to counteract hemorrhagic shock.

If needed, a single 18-gauge needle access is acceptable for fluid resuscitation. TECC caregivers are still following the damage control resuscitation protocol. If no blood products are available, crystalloid is the next fluid of choice for resuscitation. Administration of lactated Ringer or normal saline should proceed in 250-ml boluses until a palpable radial pulse is restored or systolic blood pressure is between 80 and 90 mm Hg.

> **CHECK YOUR KNOWLEDGE**
>
> **The goal of evacuation care/cold zone fluid resuscitation for patients without traumatic brain injury is to:**
>
> a. maintain a systolic blood pressure between 120 and 130 mm Hg.
> b. maintain a diastolic blood pressure between 80 and 90 mm Hg.
> c. increase the number of red blood cells.
> d. maintain a palpable radial pulse.

Evacuation Care: Traumatic Brain Injury

Traumatic brain injury (TBI) occurs when external mechanical forces impact the head and cause an acceleration/deceleration of the brain within the cranial vault that results in injury to brain tissue. A TBI may be closed (blunt or blast trauma) or open (penetrating trauma). Signs and symptoms of TBI are highly variable and depend on the specific areas of the brain affected and the injury severity. Alteration in consciousness and focal neurologic deficits are common. Various forms of intracranial hemorrhage (ICH), such as epidural hematoma, subdural hematoma, subarachnoid hemorrhage, and hemorrhagic contusion, can be components of a TBI. Moderate and severe TBIs are life-threatening injuries.

TECC caregivers need to focus on the complications, or secondary brain injuries, from a TBI:

- Brain swelling
- Rise in intracranial pressure
- Decrease in cerebral perfusion

These complications can lead to massive swelling, compression of the brain stem, and, ultimately, death.

The brain is vitally dependent on a continuous supply of oxygenated blood. When a casualty's systolic blood pressure is less than 90 mm Hg or oxygen saturation via pulse oximetry (Spo_2) is less than 90%, this more than doubles the risk of death from brain injury. This requires the TECC caregiver to manage the following:

- Hypotension: maintain blood pressure above 90 mm Hg.
- Hypoxia: keep pulse oximetry (Spo_2) above 90%.
- Hypocarbia or hypercarbia: maintain adequate ventilation to keep CO_2 levels within normal range using capnography.
- Hypoglycemia: keep blood glucose level above 70 mg/dl.

In addition, be alert for signs of elevated intracranial pressure such as a headache, blurred vision, vomiting, hypertension, shallow breathing, weakness, or problems with walking and talking, or behavioral changes.

Altered Mental Status With Suspected TBI

The initial or early signs of TBI may be subtle and relate to small increases in intracranial pressure. They include the following:

- Headache
- Nausea
- Altered level of consciousness
- Glasgow Coma Scale (GCS) score <15

If left untreated, intracranial pressure may increase and result in herniation of the brain. Assessment findings with brain herniation may include the following:

- Unilateral or bilateral pupil dilatation
- Glasgow Coma Scale score <8
- Cushing's triad (widened pulse pressure, bradycardia, irregular respirations)
- Absence of deep tendon and plantar responses
- Abnormal posturing (decorticate and decerebrate)

Initial documentation of the GCS is a vital step in the assessment process. The initial GCS will serve as a baseline on which future neurologic assessments will be based. The brief neurologic assessment in the primary survey should include not only the GCS but also the level of consciousness, pupillary size and response to light, presence of any posturing, and vital signs review. The neurologic assessment in the secondary survey can be in more detail.

Fluid Resuscitation of TBI

Hypotension and hypoxia will worsen patient outcomes if the patient also has a TBI. Appropriate fluid resuscitation can prevent the deleterious effect of an episode of hypotension in a patient with traumatic brain injury. Provide fluids to maintain a systolic blood pressure of 90 to 100 mm Hg. Assess for strong peripheral pulses and mental status. If possible, transport the patient with the head elevated 30 degrees.

> **CHECK YOUR KNOWLEDGE**
>
> _____ more than doubles the risk of death from brain injury.
>
> a. Uneven pupillary response to light
> b. Decorticate posturing
> c. Systolic blood pressure >120 mm Hg
> d. Oxygen saturation via pulse oximetry (Spo_2) <90%

Evacuation Care: Burns

Inhalation injury is a severe complication in burned individuals or victims of fires in confined spaces. One of the factors that contributes to such problems is lung dysfunction, which might rapidly lead to hard-to-manage hypoxemia and poisoning by inhaled toxic by-products, such as carbon monoxide and cyanide. Early recognition and treatment of poisoning are crucial for the patients' recovery.

At the time of the initial assessment, early intubation should be considered when signs of considerable airway swelling are present including stridor, use of accessory muscles, respiratory distress, hypoventilation, and face or neck burns. During the assessment of breathing, the Fio_2 should be kept at 100% to correct the hypoxemia resulting from the low oxygen concentration in the inspired air in fire environments.

BOX 8-1
Symptoms of Carbon Monoxide Poisoning

- **Mild**
  - Headache
  - Fatigue
  - Nausea
- **Moderate**
  - Severe headache
  - Vomiting
  - Confusion
  - Drowsiness/sleepiness
  - Increased heart rate and ventilatory rate
- **Severe**
  - Seizures
  - Coma
  - Cardiorespiratory arrest
  - Death

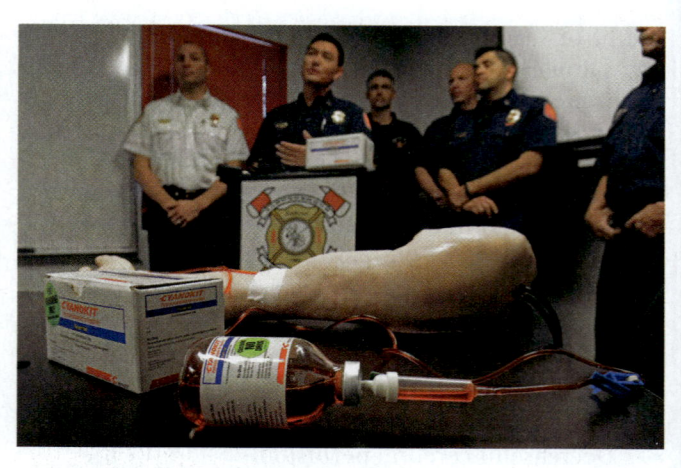

Figure 8-7 Contents of CYANOKIT.
© Jim Thompson/Albuquerque Journal/ZUMA Press Inc/Alamy Stock Photo.

CYANOKIT

CYANOKIT (hydroxocobalamin for injection) 5 g is indicated for the treatment of known or suspected cyanide poisoning. If clinical suspicion of cyanide poisoning is high, CYANOKIT should be administered without delay. Particular attention should be paid to neurologic examination because the level of consciousness is frequently reduced by hypoxemia/hypercapnia or carbon monoxide/cyanide poisoning. The starting dose of CYANOKIT for adults is 5 g (contained in a single vial), administered by IV infusion over 15 minutes (approximately 15 ml/min). Depending upon the severity of the poisoning and the clinical response, a second dose of 5 g may be administered by IV infusion up to a total dose of 10 g. The rate of infusion for a potential second dose may range from 15 minutes (for patients in extremis) to 2 hours, as clinically indicated (**Figure 8-7**).

Amyl Nitrite

Amyl nitrite, a compound that has vasodilatory properties and that oxidizes hemoglobin to cyanide-binding methemoglobin, has also been used to treat cyanide poisoning. It is often, but not always, administered with other agents (sodium nitrite and sodium thiosulfate) in a cyanide antidote kit and with other supportive measures such as oxygen.

A retrospective study examining the treatment of cyanide intoxication in industrial workers concluded that amyl nitrite was effective, with no residual adverse effects except headache and transient loss of appetite. However, other studies have cautioned about the use of amyl nitrite to treat mass-casualty cyanide poisoning due to several limitations: uncontrolled administration of amyl nitrite ampules with potential inadequate dosing; potential for serious toxicity such as nitrite-induced methemoglobinemia, and in smoke inhalation victims, carboxyhemoglobinemia with a subsequent decrease in oxygen delivery to vital tissues and organs; and distracted management by caregivers of a mass-casualty incident. Administration of amyl nitrite using a nebulizer or inhaler may help to minimize its deficiencies. In summary, studies demonstrating the safety and efficacy of amyl nitrite are inconclusive, and its risk–benefit profile may not be favorable. Hydroxocobalamin, which was approved by the Food and Drug Administration in 2006, has a more positive risk–benefit profile and is likely a better antidote for cyanide poisoning.

Sodium Thiosulfate

Sodium thiosulfate enhances the conversion of cyanide to thiocyanate, which is renally excreted. Thiosulfate has a somewhat delayed effect and thus is typically used with sodium nitrite for faster antidote action. Sodium nitrite must be used with caution because it may result in significant hypotension and cardiovascular collapse, in addition to generating dangerous levels of methemoglobin. However, in cases of smoke inhalation in which cyanide toxicity is suspected, administration of sodium thiosulfate is safe.

Example of a Hydrogen Cyanide Poisoning Protocol

1. Patients with severe exposure (unconscious, not breathing) should immediately receive 100% oxygen. Cardiac monitoring and evaluation of

oxygen saturation should be done when possible. Antidotes should be administered as soon as possible (see later). It is important to note that pulse oximeter results are completely unreliable in the setting of carbon monoxide poisoning and methemoglobinemia, which is induced by amyl nitrite or sodium nitrite therapy. Normal values for oxygen saturation in these patients can be associated with profound hypoxemia.
2. Ventilate using bag-mask device with one ampule of amyl nitrite (crushed) in bag; after several minutes add another (crushed) ampule; keep adding an ampule every several minutes. This is a temporary measure until IV medications can be given, but it may assist in recovery.
3. Administer 300 mg (10 ml) of sodium nitrite IV over 5 minutes, and then flush the line (children's dose: 0.2–0.3 ml/kg, or 6–9 mg/kg of the 3% solution). There is no separate recommendation for infants. For elderly patients, use adult dose unless small and frail. Be aware that nitrites produce orthostatic hypertension, but a patient who can stand does not need them.
4. Follow with 12.5 g (50 ml) of sodium thiosulfate IV (children's dose: 0.4 mg/kg, or 1.65 ml/kg of the 25% solution). There is no separate recommendation for infants. An adult dose should be used for elderly patients unless they are small and frail. Use care in giving nitrite in a patient with hypertension or heart disease. Amyl nitrite, sodium nitrite, and sodium thiosulfate are in the Pasadena (formerly Lilly) cyanide antidote kit, the latter two in ampules of 300 mg/10 ml and 12.5 g/50 ml. Use one-half dose in 20 minutes if no improvement. See instructions on top of antidote kit box.
5. If patient continues to remain apneic, consider intubation and continue oxygen through tube with assisted ventilation.

CHECK YOUR KNOWLEDGE

Which of these statements regarding smoke inhalation patients is true?
a. Do not intubate a soot-soaked trachea.
b. Hydroxocobalamin may be a better antidote for cyanide poisoning.
c. Sodium thiosulfate is the first IV medication to use in cyanide poisoning situations.
d. The pulse oximetry device doubles the SpO_2 value in instances of carbon monoxide poisoning.

Evacuation Care: Analgesia

Analgesia is an essential part of prehospital medicine, and its efficient provision requires specific TECC caregiver skills and knowledge. Administration of analgesics or sedative drugs may be a potential source of complications such as hypotension and respiratory depression or arrest.

The National Highway Traffic Safety Administration funded an evidence-based guideline for prehospital analgesia in trauma, using the Grading of Recommendations Assessment, Development and Evaluation (GRADE) methodology. Although the group discussed oral analgesics, and nonpharmacologic means of pain control such as distraction and splinting, they felt that for maximal impact the guideline should focus on the assessment of pain and the delivery of pharmacologic agents available in the field to ALS-level EMS providers. Based on their evidence-based recommendations, the panel developed a model EMS protocol for the management of acute traumatic pain (**Figure 8-8**).

Evacuation Care: CPR

A TECC caregiver's response to a casualty in cardiac arrest provides one of the starkest examples of the risk versus reward calculation while operating in the tactical arena. In the direct threat/hot zone, a casualty found without a pulse or respiration is triaged as deceased. If a casualty goes into cardiac arrest while in the indirect threat/warm zone, the TECC caregiver will consider bilateral needle decompression for nonbreathing and pulseless casualties with torso or polytrauma (two or more significant trauma injuries). This is to rule out tension pneumothorax as the cause of the cardiac arrest before discontinuing care.

A casualty who goes into cardiac arrest while in the evacuation/cold zone will receive the same resuscitation measures that a traumatic cardiac arrest (TCA) patient would receive outside of the tactical arena. Resuscitation research shows some success in resuscitation of TCA patients delivered to the emergency department despite not achieving restoration of spontaneous circulation (ROSC) during prehospital care.

The TECC caregiver should consider the underlying clinical cause for the cardiac arrest:

- Airway compromise
- Exsanguination
- Tension pneumothorax

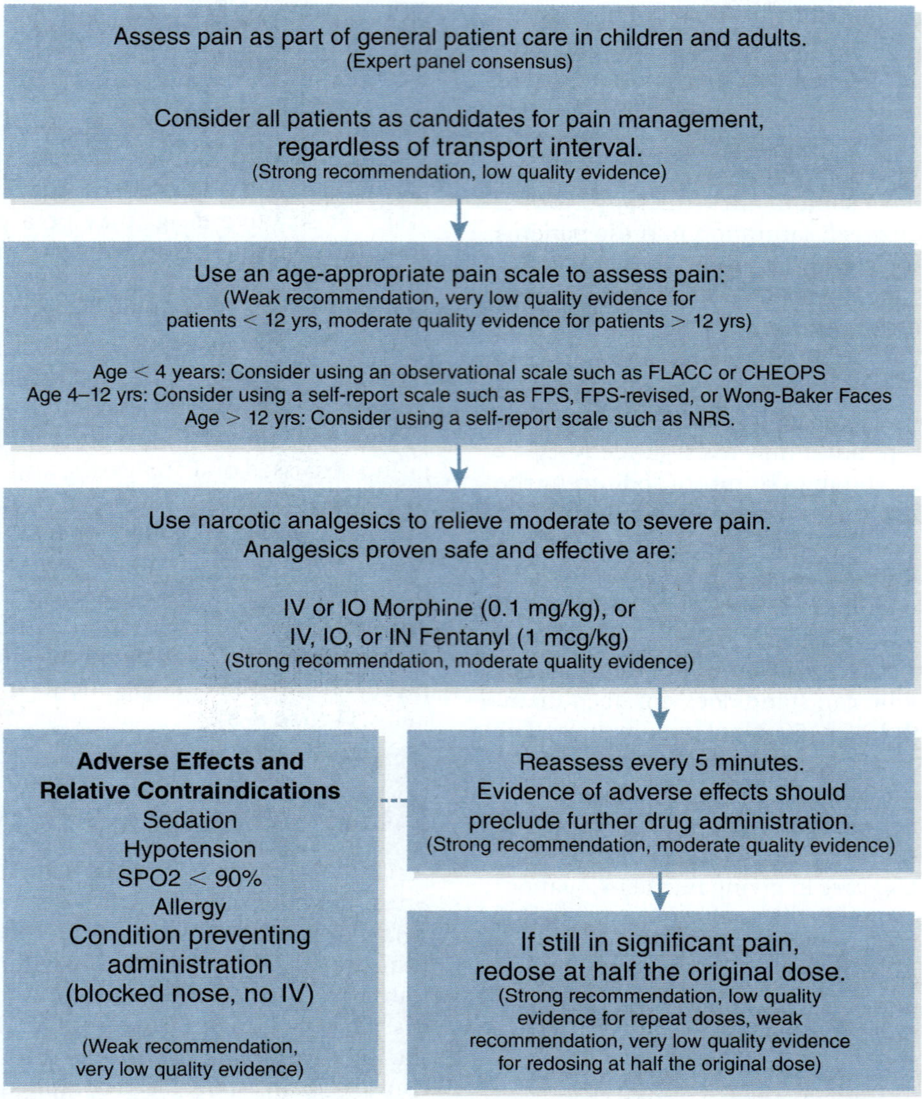

> Assess pain as part of general patient care in children and adults.
> (Expert panel consensus)
>
> Consider all patients as candidates for pain management,
> regardless of transport interval.
> (Strong recommendation, low quality evidence)
>
> Use an age-appropriate pain scale to assess pain:
> (Weak recommendation, very low quality evidence for
> patients < 12 yrs, moderate quality evidence for patients > 12 yrs)
>
> Age < 4 years: Consider using an observational scale such as FLACC or CHEOPS
> Age 4–12 yrs: Consider using a self-report scale such as FPS, FPS-revised, or Wong-Baker Faces
> Age > 12 yrs: Consider using a self-report scale such as NRS.
>
> Use narcotic analgesics to relieve moderate to severe pain.
> Analgesics proven safe and effective are:
>
> IV or IO Morphine (0.1 mg/kg), or
> IV, IO, or IN Fentanyl (1 mcg/kg)
> (Strong recommendation, moderate quality evidence)
>
> **Adverse Effects and Relative Contraindications**
> Sedation
> Hypotension
> SPO2 < 90%
> Allergy
> Condition preventing administration
> (blocked nose, no IV)
> (Weak recommendation, very low quality evidence)
>
> Reassess every 5 minutes.
> Evidence of adverse effects should preclude further drug administration.
> (Strong recommendation, moderate quality evidence)
>
> If still in significant pain, redose at half the original dose.
> (Strong recommendation, low quality evidence for repeat doses, weak recommendation, very low quality evidence for redosing at half the original dose)
>
> This protocol excludes patients who are allergic to narcotic medications and/or who have altered mentation (GCS < 15 or mentation not appropriate for age)

Figure 8-8 An evidence-based guideline for prehospital analgesia in trauma.

Reproduced with permission from Marianne Gausche-Hill, MD, Kathleen M. Brown, et. al. *An Evidence-based Guideline for Prehospital Analgesia in Trauma*, Taylor & Francis, 2013.

- Herniated brain
- Heart trauma
- Drowning
- Electrocution
- Other medical conditions

Resuscitation includes using all of the available prehospital care resources, especially items that reduce the number of caregivers working on the patient, like mechanical chest compressors.

> **CHECK YOUR KNOWLEDGE**
>
> **A cause for a traumatic cardiac arrest in the evacuation care/cold zone could be:**
>
> a. exsanguination.
> b. herniated brain.
> c. airway compromise.
> d. All of these are correct.

LESSON 8 Evacuation Care/Cold Zone

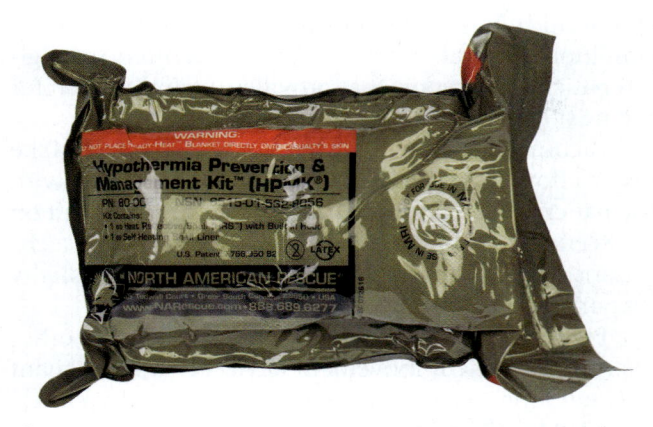

Figure 8-9 Hypothermia prevention and management kit.
Reproduced with permission from North American Rescue. Retrieved from https://www.narescue.com/nar-hypothermia-prevention-and-management-kit-hpmk

Evacuation Care: Hypothermia

Hypothermia, acidosis, and coagulopathy make up the lethal triad, a vicious cycle that leads to death in a trauma patient. Hypothermia can impact coagulation, the body's ability to form a clot. The presence of hypothermia and acidosis, which results in coagulopathy, and the relationship among these three conditions can result in a 90% death rate among victims of severe trauma.

TECC caregivers must remain vigilant to maintain the casualty's temperature while treatments are performed. The nature of certain medical conditions, the side effects of some medical interventions, and the need to expose injury sites can quickly cool the body.

TECC caregivers can counter hypothermia in trauma patients by reducing heat transfer loss by doing the following:

- Remove wet/bloody clothing.
- Cover casualties.
- Place blanket below patient.
- Transport on an insulated surface.
- Provide warm IV fluids.
- Use forced-air blanket warmers, if available.
- Use hypothermia prevention and management kits if available (**Figure 8-9**).

> ### CHECK YOUR KNOWLEDGE
> The presence of hypothermia and acidosis can result in _____ mortality in severe trauma patients.
>
> a. 90%
> b. 70%
> c. 60%
> d. 40%

Evacuation Care: Reassess, Document, Communicate, and Prepare for Movement

Preparing to move the casualty from the evacuation/cold zone is similar to moving a trauma patient outside of the tactical arena to a medical facility. TECC caregivers will perform a head-to-toe reassessment of the casualty, checking for bleeding, airway patency, and any life threats. All splints, bandages, and IV lines are reassessed.

There are two levels of documentation. One is directly on the patient for significant treatment or condition that needs to be conveyed to the receiving facility independent of paper, voice, or electronic notifications. Placement of a tourniquet and establishment of an IV line are two time-sensitive activities that need to be recorded on the patient.

The second level of documentation is the data found on a prehospital care report. Initial observation, prehospital care delivered, vital signs, and patient history are included in the prehospital care report. Due to the austere nature of tactical arenas, this documentation may be found on a triage tag (**Figure 8-10**).

Some regional and state EMS systems are using radio frequency identification (RFID) triage tags and electronic patient care reporting systems as part of a comprehensive patient tracking system that starts at the incident scene and proceeds through patient disposition.

Communicating With the Patient

In preparing for the move from the evacuation/cold zone, reassure the casualty that the situation is improving, direct the person to continue self-care, and explain where the patient is going. Your role is to be calm, clear, and consistent in message, instructions, and demeanor.

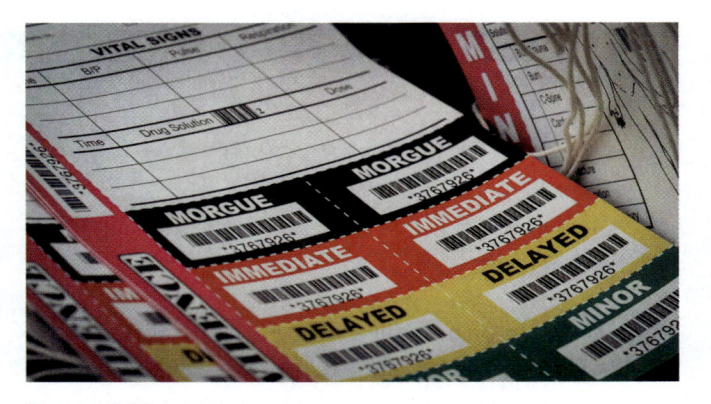

Figure 8-10 Triage tags.
© U.S. Air Force photo/ Sgt. Benjamin Raughton/Archistoric/Alamy Stock Photo.

Communicating With Receiving Hospitals

Communications from the evacuation/cold zone will vary based on the tactical arena and community resources. On one side of the spectrum, communications will be between the hospital and the transportation sector within the incident management system. That communication may be digital. In some areas there is a state or regional dispatch center that coordinates patient destinations with existing conditions using real-time bed access data from all of the receiving hospitals in the region.

In Maryland, for example, the Emergency Medical Resources Center (EMRC) coordinates medical consultation between medic units and hospital physicians. Medic units requesting a medical consult can call EMRC, where operators instruct them to switch over to an available med channel to be patched through to a hospital. While en route to the receiving hospital, prehospital providers transmit patient information to an online hospital physician. Physicians may direct the prehospital provider to follow specific medical protocols and give them approval for additional treatment.

On the other side of the spectrum, a TECC caregiver uses a radio or cellphone to alert the receiving hospital regarding each casualty leaving the evacuation/cold zone, tracked on a sheet of paper. Regardless of the technology, the hospitals need to know the number of patients, patient current conditions, and prehospital treatment.

Based on the experience of recent incidents, emergency departments may already be busy with casualties that bypassed EMS and went directly to the hospital. The goal with TECC is to get each casualty to the most appropriate hospital.

Preparing for Patient Movement

The casualty is leaving the tactical arena to be transported to a medical facility. Provide adequate verbal communications to the transport team on the patient's condition, treatment provided, and a written (or digital) patient care report that provides the foundation for the next level of care.

Tactical incidents will also be crime scenes. Make every effort to keep the patient's clothing either with the patient or document where the clothing was left on the scene. It would be helpful to the crime scene technicians to also get a description of where the casualty was originally located.

Properly secure the patient on a stretcher or other appropriate patient movement device. Remain vigilant to conditions or situations that would create hypothermia. Follow all patient safety precautions.

> **CHECK YOUR KNOWLEDGE**
>
> **Time-sensitive prehospital treatments that need to be recorded on the patient include:**
>
> a. when tourniquet was applied.
> b. size of IV cannula.
> c. initial vital signs.
> d. when rewarming efforts began.

Summary

- Have an evacuation plan.
  - Primary, secondary, and tertiary
- Reassess, reassess, reassess.
- Treat casualty.
  - Primary survey
  - Secondary survey
- Introduce electronic monitoring equipment.
- Communicate with casualties.
- Provide early notification to receiving facilities.
- Document care provided.

REFERENCES AND RESOURCES

American College of Surgeons. *Strategies to Enhance Survival and Intentional Mass Casualty Events*. Chicago: American College of Surgeons; 2015.

Ciottone GR. *Ciottone's Disaster Medicine*. 2nd ed. Atlanta, GA: Elsevier; 2015.

Drew B, Bird D, Matteucci M, Keenan S. Tourniquet conversion: a recommended approach in the prolonged field care setting. *J Spec Oper Med*. 2015;15(3):81-85.

Emergency Management Institute. *IS-907 Active Shooter: What You Can Do. Student Manual*. Washington, DC: National Protection and Programs Directorate/Office of Infrastructure Protection, U.S. Department of Homeland Security; 2015.

EMS challenges and lessons learned from the Ferguson riots. EMS1.com website. https://www.ems1.com/ems-products/communications/articles/2146450-EMS-challenges-and-lessons-learned-from-the-Ferguson-riots/. March 30, 2015.

Gausche-Hill M, Brown KM, Oliver ZJ, Sasson C, Dayan PS, Eschmann NM, Weik TS, Lawner BJ, Sahni R,

Falck-Ytter Y, Wright JL, Todd K, Lang ES. An evidence-based guideline for prehospital analgesia in trauma. *Prehosp Emerg Care*. 2014;18:(Sup1):25-34.

Haley KB, Brooke Lerner EB, Guse CE, Pirrallo RG. Effect of system-wide interventions on the assessment and treatment of pain by emergency medical services providers. *Prehosp Emerg Care*. 2016;20(6):752-758.

Holcomb, JB. Major scientific lessons learned in the trauma field over the last two decades. *PLoS Med*. 2017;14(7):e1002339.

Joint Trauma System Clinical Practice Guideline. *Traumatic Brain Injury Management in Prolonged Field Care* (CPG ID: 63). Washington, DC: Department of Defense; 2017.

Koerth-Baker M. Only 6 percent of U. S. terrorists act alone, but they are prolific. FiveThirtyEight.com website. https://fivethirtyeight.com/features/pipe-bomb-lone-wolf-terrorism/. October 26, 2018.

National Association of Emergency Medical Technicians. *PHTLS: Prehospital Trauma Life Support*. 9th ed. Burlington, MA: Public Safety Group; 2019.

Office of Health Affairs. *First Responder Guide for Improving Survivability in Improvised Explosive Device and/or Active Shooter Incidents*. Washington: DC: Department of Homeland Security; 2015.

Phillips PJ. Lone wolf terrorism. *Peace Econ Peace Sci Pub Pol*. 2011;17(1):1-29.

Ramesh AC, Kumar S. Triage, monitoring, and treatment of mass casualty events involving chemical, biological, radiological, or nuclear agents. *J Pharm Bioallied Sci*. 2010;2(3):239-247.

Roberts I, Prieto-Merino D, Manno D. Mechanism of action of tranexamic acid in bleeding trauma patients: an exploratory analysis of data from the CRASH-2 trial. *Crit Care (London, England)*. 2014;18(6):685.

Snyder D, Tsou A, Schoelles K. *Efficacy of Prehospital Application of Tourniquets and Hemostatic Dressings to Control Traumatic External Hemorrhage*. Washington, DC: National Highway Traffic Safety Administration; 2014.

Spaaj R. The enigma of lone wolf terrorism: an assessment. *Stud Conflict Terror*. 2010;33(9):854-870.

Takesh N, Kinoshita T, Yamakawa K. Tranexamic acid and trauma-induced coagulopathy. *J Intens Care*. 2017;5:5.

U.S. Army Training and Doctrine Command. *A Military Guide to Terrorism in the Twenty-First Century* (Version 5.0). Fort Leavenworth, KS: TRADOC Army Training and Doctrine Command; 2007.

LESSON 9

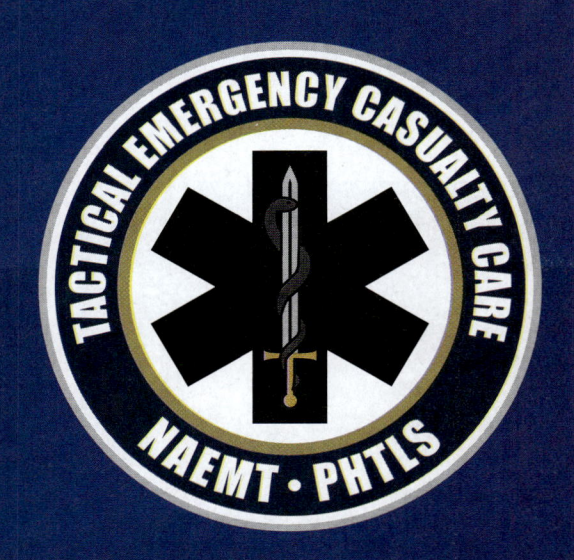

Triage

LESSON OBJECTIVES
- Discuss the difference between primary and secondary triage.
- Identify the limitations to current triage algorithms.
- Explain how triage is impacted when resources are limited.

Overview of TECC Triage

Lesson 9: Triage takes a detailed look at triage systems and limitations when operating in the tactical arena.

Triage Concepts

Triage is a French word meaning "to sort." Triage is a process that is used to assign priority for treatment and transport. In the prehospital environment, triage is used in two different contexts:

1. Sufficient resources are available to manage all patients. In this triage situation, the most severely injured patients are treated and transported first, and those with lesser injuries are treated and transported later.
2. The number of patients exceeds the immediate capacity of on-scene resources. The objective in such triage situations is to ensure survival of the largest possible number of injured patients. Patients are sorted into categories for patient care. In a mass-casualty incident (MCI), patient care must be rationed because the number of patients exceeds the available resources.

Relatively few prehospital care providers ever experience an MCI with 50 to 100 or more simultaneously injured persons, but many will be involved in MCIs with 10 to 20 patients, and most prehospital care providers have managed an incident with 2 to 10 patients. The Centers for Disease Control and Prevention (CDC) defines a mass-casualty event as usually involving six or more casualties.

The goal of patient management at the MCI scene is to do the most good for the most patients with the resources available. It is the responsibility of the tactical emergency casualty care (TECC) caregiver to make decisions about who will be managed first. The usual rules about saving lives are different in MCIs. The decision is always to save the most lives; however, when the available resources are not sufficient for the needs of all the injured patients present, these resources should be used for the patients who have the best chance of surviving.

In a choice between a patient with a catastrophic injury, such as severe brain trauma, and a patient with acute intra-abdominal hemorrhage, the proper course of action in an MCI is to first manage the salvageable patient—the patient with the intra-abdominal hemorrhage. Treating the patient with severe head trauma first will probably result in the loss of both patients; the head trauma patient may die because he or she may not be salvageable, and the intra-abdominal hemorrhage patient may die because time, equipment, and EMS personnel spent managing the unsalvageable patient kept this salvageable patient from receiving the simple care needed to survive until definitive surgical care was available.

In a triage MCI situation, the catastrophically injured patient may need to be considered "lower priority," with treatment delayed until more help and equipment become available. These are difficult decisions and circumstances, but TECC providers must respond quickly and properly. TECC caregivers with few resources should not make efforts to resuscitate a traumatic cardiac arrest patient with little chance of survival while three other patients die because of exsanguinating external hemorrhage. The "sorting scheme" most often used divides patients into five categories based on need of care and chance of survival:

1. Immediate—Patients whose injuries are critical, but who will require only minimal time or equipment to manage and who have a good prognosis for survival. An example is the patient with a compromised airway or massive external hemorrhage.
2. Delayed—Patients whose injuries are debilitating, but who do not require immediate management to salvage life or limb. An example is the patient with a long-bone fracture.
3. Minor—Patients, often called the "walking wounded," who have minor injuries that can wait for treatment or who may even assist in the interim by comforting other patients or helping as litter bearers.
4. Expectant—Patients whose injuries are so severe that they have only a minimal chance of survival. An example is the patient with a 90% full-thickness burn and thermal pulmonary injury.
5. Dead—Patients who are unresponsive, pulseless, and breathless. In a disaster, resources rarely allow for attempted resuscitation of cardiac arrest patients.

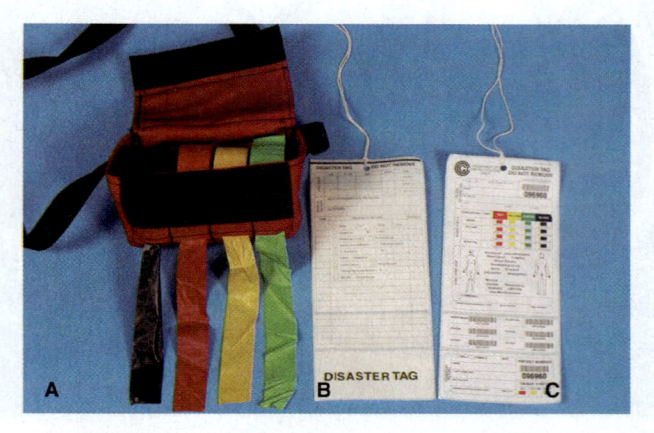

Figure 9-1 Triage tags (from left to right). **A.** Waterproof weapons of mass destruction tape. **B.** Triage tag: back. **C.** Triage tag: front.
© Jones & Bartlett Learning.

The main information needed on the tag is a unique number and a triage category. Rapid and accurate triage will help bring order to the chaos of the MCI scene and allow the most critical patients to be transported first. After the primary triage the TECC caregiver should communicate the following information to the sector supervisor, medical branch manager, or incident commander:

- The total number of patients
- The number of patients in each of the triage categories
- Recommendations for extrication and movement of patients to the treatment area
- Resources needed to complete triage and begin movement of patients to the evacuation/cold zone sector

> **CHECK YOUR KNOWLEDGE**
>
> **A casualty triaged as _____ may be engaged as a patient mover.**
>
> a. immediate
> b. delayed
> c. minor
> d. expectant

> **CHECK YOUR KNOWLEDGE**
>
> **A main activity in primary triage is to:**
>
> a. document baseline vital signs on each patient.
> b. document the triage classification on each patient.
> c. determine the number of guns and caliber of weapons in use.
> d. determine the level of chemical exposure.

Primary Triage

Primary triage is the first assessment done by the TECC caregiver to quickly and accurately categorize the patient's condition and transport needs. Primary triage can be started once the casualties are off the "X" and out of the direct threat/hot zone. During primary triage, patients are briefly assessed and then identified in some way, usually by attaching a triage tag or triage tape (**Figure 9-1**).

Limitations of Triage Systems

In an international study of triage systems, David C. Cone and Kristi L. Koenig concluded "Currently, there are many trauma triage schemes in use throughout the world. Few of these, however, are intended for mass casualty triage in the sorting and prioritizing of multiple patients at a mass casualty incident or disaster." They further noted that in-field triage is intended to allow prehospital personnel to determine whether a single given patient requires the resources of a trauma center.

Most analysis of triage systems is based on simulations and mass-casualty drills. Mass-casualty tactical incidents in Boston, Orlando, and Las Vegas reinforce the limits of all triage systems. Even with those limitations, utilizing a triage system to count the number of casualties and the level of priority is vital. The triage report guides the incident commander and medical community in assembling appropriate resources to handle the casualties coming from the tactical arena.

> **CHECK YOUR KNOWLEDGE**
>
> **A critique of triage systems:**
>
> a. focuses on identifying individuals needing a trauma center.
> b. identifies the number of casualties and level of priority.
> c. provides a scope of the incident to the incident commander.
> d. provides earliest notice of transport requirements.

START Triage

START triage is one of the easiest methods of triage. START stands for Simple Triage And Rapid Treatment. The staff members at Hoag Memorial Hospital, Newport Beach, CA, were responsible for developing this method of triage in 1983. START triage uses a limited assessment of the patient's ability to walk, respiratory status, hemodynamic status (pulse), and neurologic status. (**Figure 9-2**).

The first step of the START triage system is performed on arrival at the scene by calling out to patients at the disaster site, "If you can hear my voice and are able to walk . . ." and then directing patients to an easily identifiable landmark. The injured persons in this group are the walking wounded and are considered minimal (green) priority, or third-priority patients. In the tactical arena, do not have casualties walk through the direct threat/hot zone.

The second step in the START process is directed toward nonwalking patients. Move to the first nonambulatory patient and assess the respiratory status. If the patient is not breathing, open the airway by using a simple manual maneuver. A patient who still does not begin to breathe is triaged as expectant (black). If the patient begins to breathe, tag him or her as immediate (red) and place in the recovery position and move on to the next patient.

If the patient is breathing, a quick estimation of the respiratory rate should be made. A patient who is breathing faster than 30 breaths/min or slower than 10 breaths/min is triaged as an immediate priority (red). If the patient is breathing from 10 to 29 breaths/min, move to the next step of the assessment.

The next step is to assess the hemodynamic status of the patient by checking for bilateral radial pulses. An absent radial pulse implies the patient is hypotensive and should be triaged as an immediate priority. If the radial pulse is present, go to the next assessment.

The final assessment in START triage is to assess the patient's neurologic status, which simply means to assess the patient's ability to follow simple commands, such as "show me three fingers." This assessment establishes that the patient can understand and follow commands. A patient who is unconscious or cannot follow simple commands is an immediate priority patient. A patient who complies with a simple command should be triaged in the delayed category.

> **CHECK YOUR KNOWLEDGE**
>
> **A patient who is breathing faster than 30 breaths/min is triaged as:**
>
> a. immediate.
> b. delayed.
> c. Imminent.
> d. minor.

SALT Triage

In 2012 the CDC released a report titled "Guidelines for Field Triage of Injured Patients, Recommendations of a National Expert Panel on Field Triage." This document revisited the 1986 ACS Field Triage Decision Scheme; it also looked at all of the data posted since the last workgroup meeting in 2006. The SALT triage scheme was intended to develop a methodology that would be the basis for a national triage system for MCIs following the science and consensus-based Model Uniform Core Criteria (MUCC) (**Figure 9-3**).

The Sort, Assess, Lifesaving interventions, and Treatment and/or Transport (SALT) triage system begins by using a global sorting of patients. This first step identifies the patients who are able to understand verbal instructions and are therefore likely to have

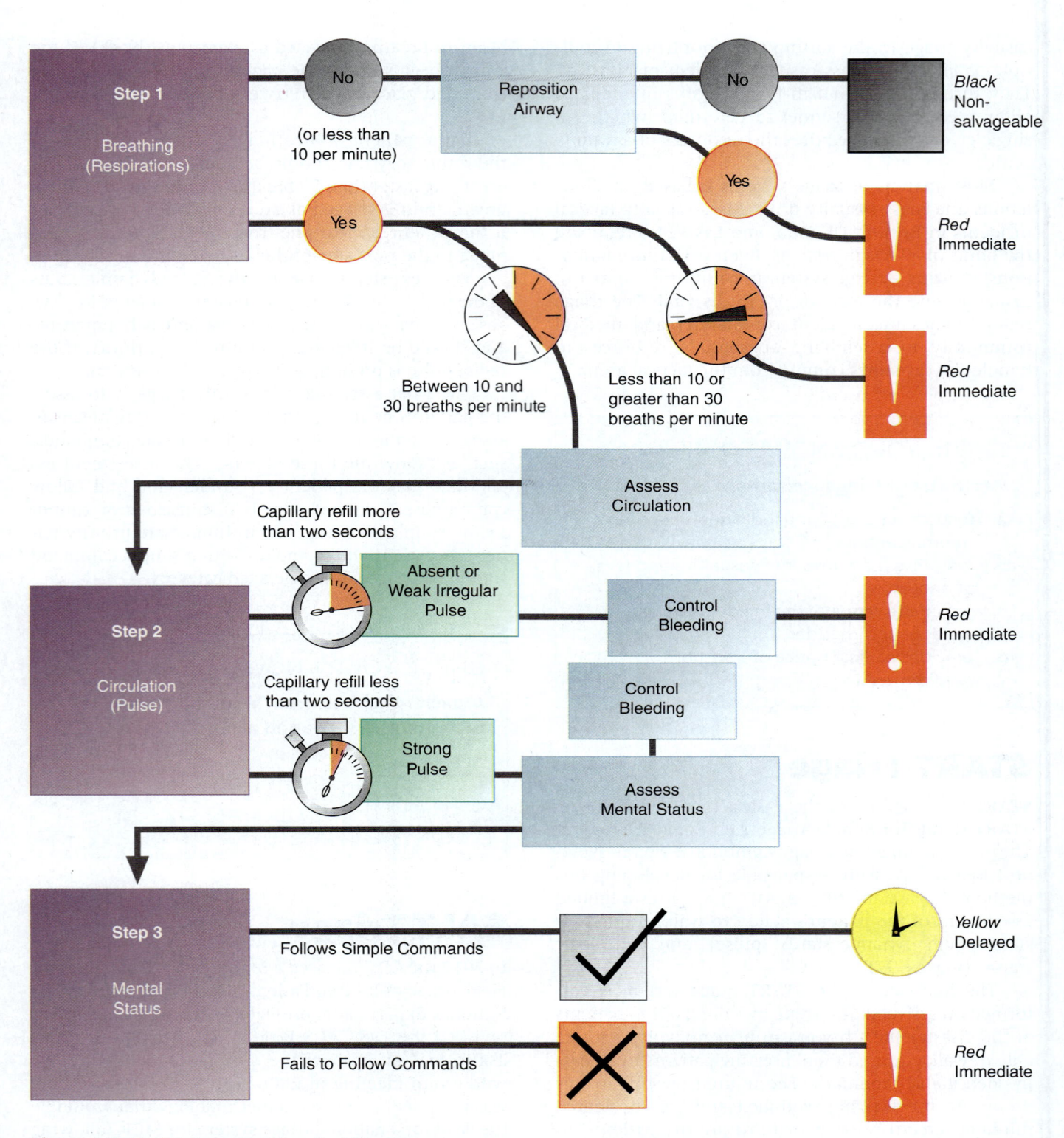

Figure 9-2 START triage algorithm decision map.
Courtesy of Hoag Hospital Newport Beach and the Newport Beach Fire Department.

good perfusion. These patients are given a collection point to move to for further instructions. This is an attempt to decrease the number of patients leaving the scene and overwhelming local hospital resources before EMS can begin to move the highest priority patients. The SALT method differs from others in its lifesaving intervention steps, which include bleeding control, opening the airway, two rescue breaths for children, needle decompression for tension pneumothorax, and autoinjector antidotes. The START method uses respirations, pulse, and neurologic status to assign priority.

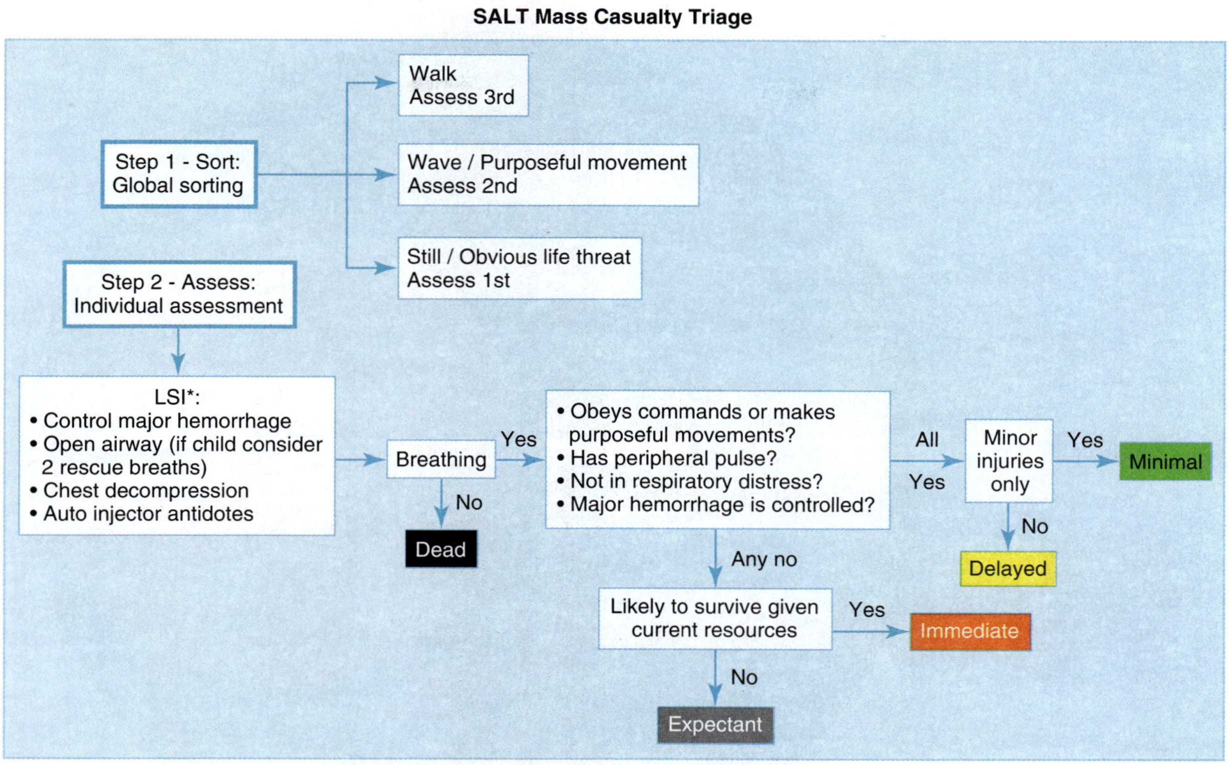

SALT Mass Casualty Triage

Figure 9-3 SALT mass-casualty algorithm.
Chemical Hazards Emergency Medical Management, U.S. Department of Health and Human Services. http://chemm.nlm.nih.gov/chemmimages/salt.png. Accessed October 16, 2017.

Numerous studies have been done on the different triage systems since START in 1983; however, no empirical evidence has proven one system to be the best. Due to the fact that communities will choose what is best for their first responders there has been no consensus on one national triage system.

> **CHECK YOUR KNOWLEDGE**
>
> **In what way does the SALT method differ from other triage systems?**
>
> a. Utilization of on-line medical control
> b. Use of lifesaving steps as part of triage assessment
> c. Focusing on patients who can wave but not walk
> d. Faster processing of patients to the transport section

Sacco Triage Method

ThinkSharp Inc. developed a commercial, evidence-based, and outcome-driven approach called the Sacco Triage Method (STM). STM uses a simple physiologic score that predicts survival and deterioration, where patients are triaged to maximize expected survivors in consideration of the timing and availability of transport and resources.

In addition to the START and STM triage systems having been derived using markedly different methods, an important difference between the two triage methods is that the START system is open-source and in the public domain, while the STM system is proprietary and licensed for commercial use only. According to a 2016 study by Jain, Ragazzoni, Stryhn, Stratton, and Corte, a trial comparing the START and Sacco triage systems used by 26 advanced care paramedic students triaging 10 patients found no statistically significant difference in total triage times.

Secondary Triage Decisions

Secondary triage in the tactical arena occurs in the indirect threat/warm zone as TECC caregivers are organizing the transfer of casualties to the evacuation/cold zone (**Figure 9-4**). The immediate tactical situation and patient response to treatment guide the secondary triage decisions.

Tactical Situation

- Has a secure corridor been established to move casualties from indirect threat/warm zone care to evacuation/cold zone care?
- How many casualties are moving to evacuation/cold zone care?

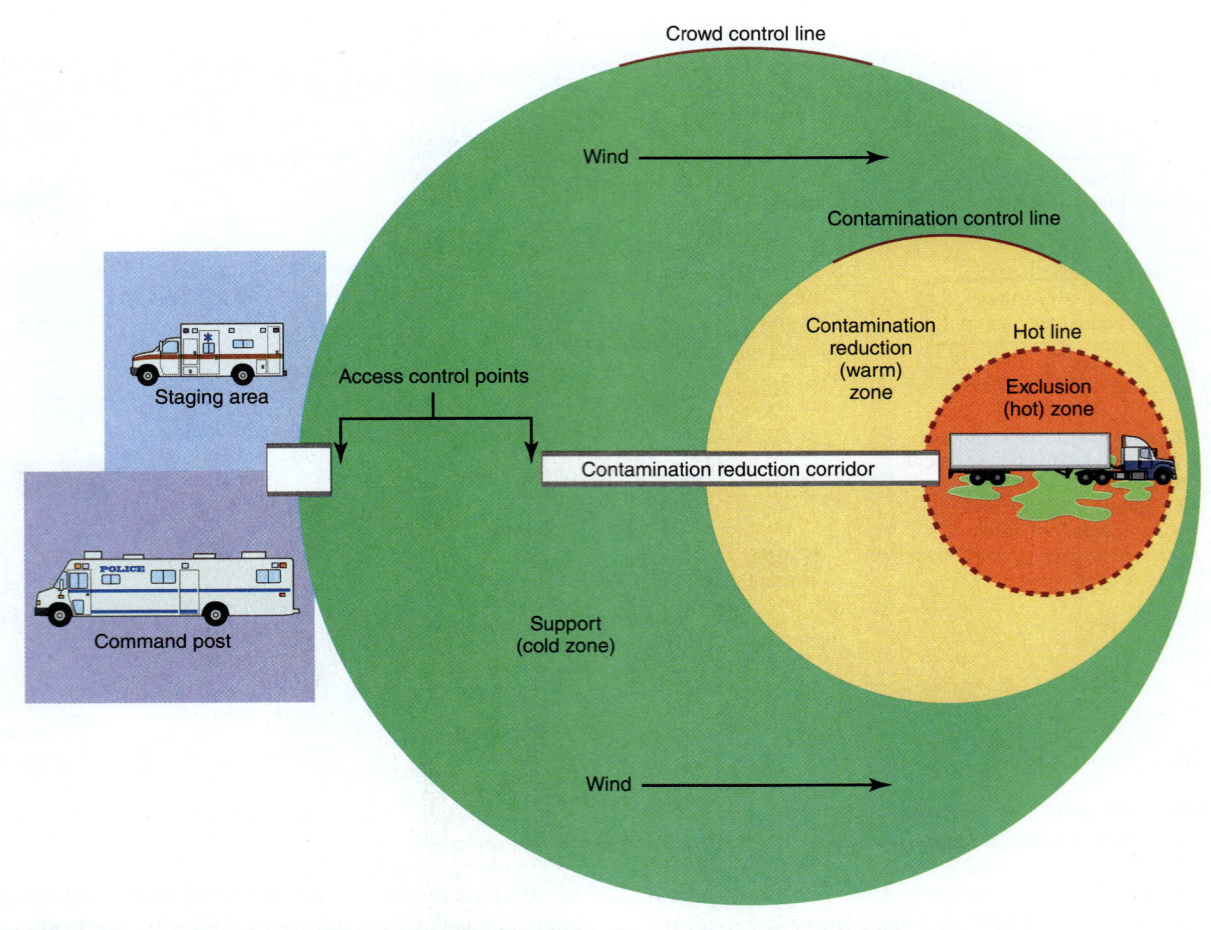

Figure 9-4 The scene of an incident is generally divided into hot, warm, and cold zones.
© National Association of Emergency Medical Technicians (NAEMT).

- How many casualties need to be carried?
- What human and technical resources are available to move patients?
- Based on latest situational awareness, how long will the corridor remain secure?

Casualty Response to MARCH Treatments

The secondary triage also checks on the effectiveness of MARCH treatments provided in the indirect threat/warm zone. Maintaining the goal of doing the most good for the most patients with the resources available means the secondary triage will establish the order of patients moved to the evacuation/cold zone.

The evacuation/cold zone will have more resources and caregivers capable of providing advanced prehospital care, which the community provides outside of the tactical arena. When retriaging casualties, consider those who will immediately benefit from prehospital care such as aggressive fluid resuscitation or who need more definitive care to handle a medical situation like diabetic ketoacidosis.

> **CHECK YOUR KNOWLEDGE**
>
> **Secondary triage includes analysis of _____ and _____.**
>
> a. anticipated tactical situation; patient response to MARCH treatments
> b. immediate tactical situation; patient vital signs
> c. projected tactical situation; patient vital signs
> d. immediate tactical situation; patient response to MARCH treatments

Summary

- Tactical situations present unique challenges as providers attempt to triage patients.
- In addition to sorting casualties, lifesaving interventions should be applied per the MARCH algorithm.
- Algorithmic sorting of casualties is a good baseline but not a substitute for provider intuition and experience.

REFERENCES AND RESOURCES

Auf der Heide E. The importance of evidence-based disaster planning. *Ann Emerg Med.* 2006;47(1):34-49.

Cone DC, Koenig KL. Mass casualty triage in the chemical, biological, or nuclear environment. *Eur J Emerg Med.* 2005;12(6):287-302.

Federal Emergency Management Agency. *1 October After-Action Report.* Washington DC: FEMA. https://www.hsdl.org/?view&did=814668. August 24, 2018.

Jain TN, Ragazzoni L, Stryhn H, Stratton SJ, Corte D. Comparison of the Sacco Triage Method versus START triage using a virtual reality scenario in advance care paramedic students. *Canad J Emerg Med.* 2016;18(4):288-292.

Leonard HB, Cole CM, Howitt AM, Heymann PB. *Why Was Boston Strong? Lessons from the Boston Marathon Bombing.* Cambridge MA: Harvard Kennedy School; 2014.

Lerner EB, McKee CH, Cady CE, et al. A consensus-based gold standard for the evaluation of mass casualty triage systems. *Prehosp Emerg Care.* 2015;19(2):267-271.

National Association of Emergency Medical Technicians. *PHTLS: Prehospital Trauma Life Support.* 9th ed. Burlington, MA: Public Safety Group; 2019.

Navin DM, Sacco WJ, Waddel, R. Operational comparison of the simple triage and rapid treatment method and the Sacco Triage Method in mass casualty exercises. *J Trauma Inj Infect Crit Care.* 2010;69(1):215-225.

Timbie JW, Ringel JS, Fox DS, Waxman DA, Pillemer F, Carey C, Moore M, Karir V, Johnson TJ, Iyer N, Hu J, Shanman R, Larkin JW, Timmer M, Motala A, Perry TR, Newberry S, Kellermann AL. Allocation of scarce resources during mass casualty events. *Evid Rep Technol Assess* (Full Rep). 2012;(207):1-305.

LESSON 10

Summation

LESSON OBJECTIVES
- Discuss the importance of immediate responders.
- Review the phases of tactical emergency casualty care (TECC).
- Review direct threat care/hot zone primary goals.
- Review indirect threat care/warm zone primary goals.
- Review evacuation care/cold zone primary goals.
- Review triage.

Overview of Summation Lesson

This lesson reviews the important take-aways from each aspect of tactical emergency casualty care (TECC), from the primary goals of the direct threat care/hot zone to the medical care that can be performed in the evacuation care/cold zone.

Importance of Immediate Responders

One of the essential lessons learned is the impact of immediate responders on the survival of casualties from hemorrhage. Responders can be civilians who provide care based on community trainings such as a "Stop the Bleed" program or simply by following directions from an emergency medical dispatcher.

Law enforcement response to the incident, eliminating or isolating the threat, will prevent additional casualties while clearing the direct threat/hot zone. As immediate responders, law enforcement should be trained to provide hemorrhage control to casualties and other first responders. Likewise, special weapons and tactics (SWAT) operators should be trained in self-aid/buddy aid and may need to secure areas for other unarmed medical personnel.

TECC caregivers' first responsibility is to ensure scene safety. They may be the first medical care providers to reach casualties in the impact area, but they must make sure they do not become one of the casualties.

EMS responders who are not part of a rescue task force or SWAT team will focus on casualty evacuation. They will continue the patient care initiated by the TECC caregivers or others working in the indirect threat care/warm zone (**Figure 10-1**).

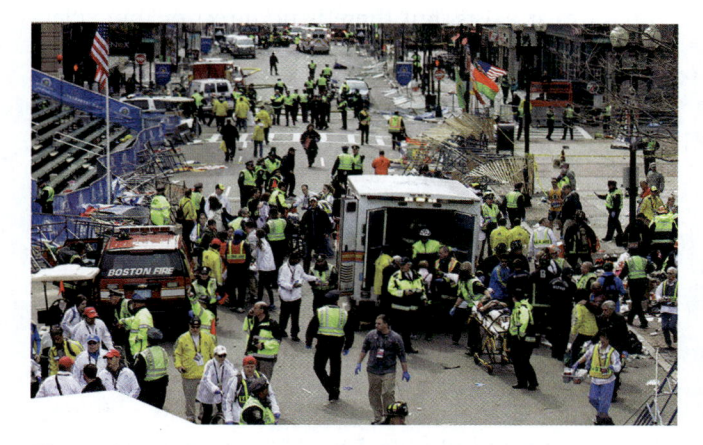

Figure 10-1 Boston Marathon patients moving to evacuation.
© Charles Krupa/AP Images.

> **CHECK YOUR KNOWLEDGE**
> **TECC caregivers' first responsibility is:**
> a. rapid assessment of patients in direct threat/hot zone.
> b. triage of patients in indirect threat/warm zone.
> c. scene safety.
> d. medical oversight of buddy-care and self-care efforts.

> **CHECK YOUR KNOWLEDGE**
> **The MARCH algorithm is exercised in the _____ zone.**
> a. hot
> b. transitional
> c. warm
> d. evacuation

Phases of TECC Care

TECC divides patient care into three zones that match the disaster management and EMS identification of caregiver and patient risk. Each zone has specific treatment goals, caregiver skills, and patient management objectives. Casualty scenarios in dynamic events usually entail both a medical problem and a tactical problem. The TECC goal is: Right Patient—Right Time—Right Care.

Direct Threat/Hot Zone

This zone represents the highest danger to caregiver and patient, as there is an immediate threat of additional injury or death because the incident scene is not secure. The emphasis in this zone is on threat suppression, preventing further casualties, extracting casualties from the high-threat area, and implementing control of life-threatening extremity hemorrhage.

Indirect Threat/Warm Zone

The indirect threat/warm zone is the area where a potential threat exists, but there is no direct or immediate threat. Indirect threat/warm zone care includes the other lifesaving interventions associated with applying the MARCH algorithm (**M**assive hemorrhage, **A**irway, **R**espiration, **C**irculation, and **H**ypothermia/**H**ead injury). Casualty collection points and rescue task forces are typically employed within the indirect threat/warm zone. The indirect threat/warm zone may return to a direct threat/hot zone situation if the threat changes or amplifies.

Evacuation Care/Cold Zone

The evacuation care/cold zone is the area where no significant threat is reasonably anticipated, and additional medical/transport resources may be staged. Evacuation/cold zone care generally falls under established local, regional, or state protocols. Most typically, this is conventional EMS/ambulance care, though it may be performed on unconventional platforms.

Direct Threat Care/Hot Zone Goals

Operating in the direct threat/hot zone is the most dangerous and dynamic zone. According to the Committee for TECC (C-TECC), the direct threat care/hot zone goals are as follows:

1. Accomplish the mission with minimal casualties.
2. Prevent any casualty from sustaining additional injuries.
3. Keep the response team maximally engaged in neutralizing the existing threat (e.g., active shooter).
4. Minimize public harm.

The priority during direct threat/hot zone care is threat suppression. Law enforcement's first goal is to stop the threat. These law enforcement officers may literally have to step over casualties in need of care in order to engage, eliminate, or confine the threat. TECC caregivers must be mindful to get off the "X" and get cover when they are in the direct threat/hot zone. If the scene is safe, they will be moving casualties off the X as quickly as possible and seeking cover. As part of remote assessment, encourage casualties who can move to get off the X.

Rapid and Remote Assessment Methodology

The purpose of the rapid and remote assessment methodology (RAM) is to maximize the opportunity to extract and treat a salvageable casualty while minimizing risk to TECC providers from attempting an unnecessary rescue.

The first step in conducting a RAM is to determine if the area is secure. If it is, standard emergency medical services (EMS) care is appropriate after ensuring that the casualty cannot harm TECC providers. If the area is not secure, use available resources (intelligence) to determine whether the casualty is a perpetrator or otherwise represents a threat. Remote observation is the first technique to be employed during the RAM because it allows providers to gather information without revealing their position. For example, a good pair of binoculars can often help to ascertain if the casualty is breathing, the rate and quality of respiration, the presence of life-threatening hemorrhage, and the presence of obvious wounds incompatible with life.

If the casualty appears stable, self-care instructions and reassurance should be communicated to the casualty, if possible, and medical extraction should await an improvement in the tactical situation. If the casualty is unstable, the risk of extraction must be weighed against the benefits of immediate access to medical care.

The casualty or person next to the casualty must first treat any life-threatening injuries with emergency interventions, such as applying tourniquets, opening the airway, and/or occluding open chest wounds as needed.

Stop the Bleeding

Control of compressible external hemorrhage during tactical field care is critical. Compressible severe external hemorrhage can usually be quickly controlled and should be the priority. Tourniquets are the first-line treatment of choice for potentially life-threatening extremity hemorrhage when and where application is possible. Any tourniquet placed on an extremity during the direct threat/hot zone phase should remain in place until the casualty arrives at the treatment hospital, unless that time will be substantially in excess of two hours in which case the tourniquet should be reevaluated to determine the need for its continued use.

Tourniquets placed to control extremity bleeding should be placed "high and tight" in the groin or armpit above the injury, directly on the skin and free of any clothing. It should be placed as snugly as possible, with as much slack removed from the tail as possible before the windlass is tightened. In the event that one tourniquet does not stop the bleeding, it is acceptable and highly recommended to use additional tourniquets side by side until bleeding is controlled, as this provides compression of the artery over a wider area.

Drags and Carries

The primary tactical goal is to get casualties off the X and into the indirect threat/warm zone. If casualties can move themselves, the TECC caregiver should direct them to the indirect threat/warm zone. This may occur while the TECC caregiver is providing remote casualty assessment where he or she cannot get to the casualty's location.

Extraction is the removal of the casualty from the direct threat/hot zone to the indirect threat/warm zone. Casualty extraction is a physically demanding process that interrupts mission flow and potentially places a tactical team in jeopardy during the extraction process from exposure to hostile fire while in a vulnerable situation dealing with a casualty.

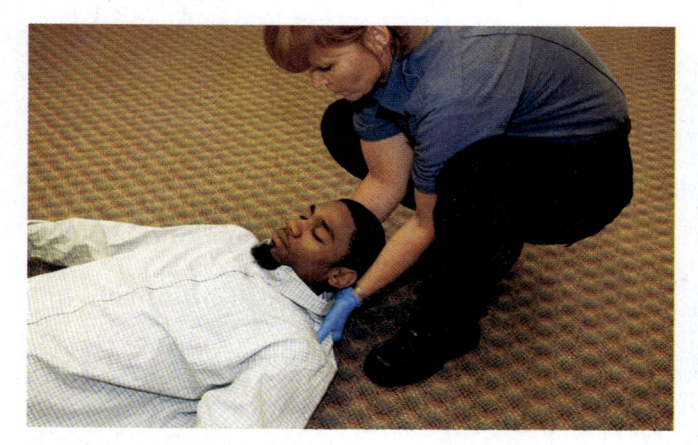

Figure 10-2 One-person drag.
© Jones & Bartlett Learning. Courtesy of MIEMSS.

Prior to extracting any casualty, the TECC provider should analyze the transit risk and likelihood of casualty survival. The time required to move a casualty is influenced by the ability of the casualty to assist, the distance involved, the casualty's gear load, relative threat levels of the area, and physical fitness of the team. If casualties cannot move themselves, drags and carries are employed to rapidly remove them from immediate danger. Common lifts, drags, and carries (LDC) include (**Figure 10-2**):

- Two-person fore/aft
- Two-person side-by-side carry
- Traditional one-person "fireman" carry
- Two-person body drag
- One-person drag
- Pack strap/Hawes carry

> **CHECK YOUR KNOWLEDGE**
>
> **The primary medical priority in the direct threat/hot zone is:**
>
> a. assure patent airway.
> b. complete initial triage.
> c. stop compressible hemorrhage.
> d. complete RAM assessment.

Indirect Threat Care/ Warm Zone Goals

Threat levels in the indirect threat care/warm zone phase vary significantly, mandating a flexible and fluid medical response. The indirect threat care/warm zone goals, according to C-TECC, are as follows:

1. Maintain operational control to stabilize the immediate scenario.
2. Conduct dedicated patient assessment and initiate appropriate lifesaving interventions.
3. *Do not delay* patient extraction/evacuation for nonlifesaving interventions.
4. Consider establishing a patient/casualty collection point.

Indirect Threat Care/Warm Zone Triage

Unless the TECC caregiver is in a fixed patient collection point, triage in the indirect threat/warm zone is significantly limited and should proceed as follows:

- Uninjured or minimally injured
  - Capable of self-care and movement
  - Need for secondary triage
- Deceased/expectant
  - Consider bilateral needle chest decompression for casualties in cardiac arrest.
- All others
  - Immediate (red tag). Patients whose injuries are critical, but who will require only minimal time or equipment to manage and who have a good prognosis for survival. An example is a patient with a compromised airway or massive external hemorrhage.
  - Delayed (yellow tag). Patients whose injuries are debilitating, but who do not require immediate management to salvage life or limb. An example is a patient with a long-bone fracture.

During triage, remove and secure all weapons from casualties with an altered mental status. During the haze of confusion after a tactical event, an armed responder suffering from a traumatic brain injury, hypoxia, or hemorrhagic shock may perceive TECC caregiver actions as an immediate life threat and aggressively respond. Weapon types include ballistic, bladed, percussion, and explosive. Consider law enforcement or military assistance to secure the weapons.

Establish communication with unified command or your designated sector officer to request patient evacuation. At this time, report the number of casualties by triage designation (red, yellow, green) and any special equipment or continuing treatment that will be required.

Developing the evacuation plan will include the route, a PACE contingency plan to cover the safe routes of travel, and the number of casualties that will need to be carried on a litter.

The indirect threat/warm zone may be part of a crime scene. Make a reasonable effort to retain casualty clothes and their initial location in the tactical arena. Preserve evidence.

Complete documentation of your patient assessment and treatment on the triage tag, directly on the patient, or in the electronic or paper-based patient flow system used by the locality.

CHECK YOUR KNOWLEDGE

The primary medical priority in the indirect threat/warm zone is:

a. *do not delay* patient extraction/evacuation for nonlifesaving interventions.
b. stage patient extraction/evacuation until the patient is stabilized and documented.
c. develop patient extrication schedule with the operational medical director or command physician.
d. develop transportation schedule with the transportation section.

Indirect Threat Care/Warm Zone: Bleeding Control

Reassess the bleeding control efforts completed in the direct threat/hot zone. Complete a head-to-toe survey blood rake-and-sweep and identify all hemorrhagic sources. Direct pressure can be used as a temporary measure.

A tourniquet remains the best choice in slowing down the progression of hemorrhagic shock and exsanguination. TECC caregivers need to assess the effectiveness of the tourniquet after every patient movement, as well as during head-to-toe reassessments. There may be a need to add a second tourniquet if the first one is ineffective.

Hemostatic dressings demonstrate successful bleeding control in injuries that are not amenable to tourniquet use. These agents have physical properties that allow the agent to adhere to damaged tissue and seal ruptured blood vessels or enhance natural blood clotting mechanisms to accelerate clot formation and produce a strengthened clot (**Figure 10-3**). After application of any of these dressings, 3 minutes of firm direct pressure should be applied. Providers should not use older powder- or granule-type agents, as they have been shown to cause thermal burns, foreign body emboli, and endothelial (internal lining of blood vessels) toxicity. Instead, using a packable hemostatic-impregnated gauze is recommended for wounds to transition zones (i.e., neck, axilla, and groin). The use of hemostatic agents must be approved in advance by the provider's medical director.

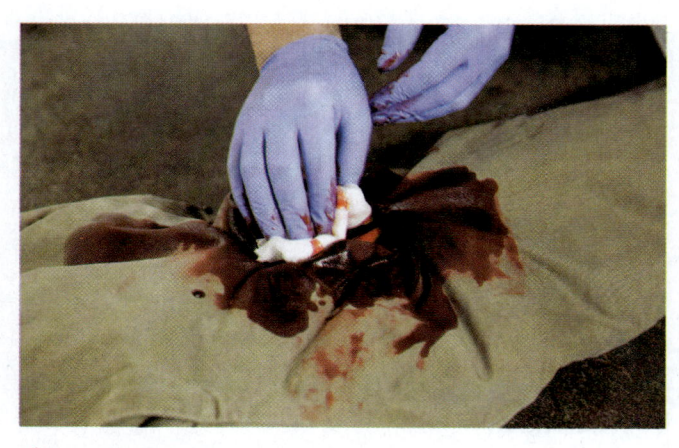

Figure 10-3 Proper packing of wound.
© Jones & Bartlett Learning. Photographed by Darren Stahlman.

Junctional tourniquets may help control hemorrhage in the groin, buttocks, perineum, axilla, and base of the neck. Tranexamic acid (TXA) can be administered intravenously, by mouth, or directly on a wound to counteract hemorrhagic shock by controlling internal bleeding. TXA should be administered based on local protocols and as soon as possible, but no later than 3 hours after the casualty was wounded.

> **CHECK YOUR KNOWLEDGE**
>
> **Control of hemorrhage in the groin, buttock, and axilla is accomplished using:**
>
> a. junctional tourniquets.
> b. tranexamic acid.
> c. both junctional tourniquets and tranexamic acid.
> d. neither junctional tourniquets nor tranexamic acid.

Indirect Threat Care/Warm Zone: Airway Control

Once major hemorrhage is controlled, the TECC caregiver looks to establish and maintain a patent airway. If the patient is conscious and able to follow commands, allow the patient to assume any position of comfort. Do not force the patient to lie down. If the patient is unconscious, or conscious but unable to follow commands, caregivers should follow this procedure:

1. Apply trauma jaw thrust maneuver to open airway.
2. Clear mouth of any foreign bodies (vomit, food, broken teeth, gum, etc.).
3. Consider placing a nasopharyngeal airway.
4. Place patient in the recovery position to maintain the open airway.
5. If the patient is unable to spontaneously maintain an open airway and adequately ventilate, use an oropharyngeal or nasopharyngeal airway and a bag-mask device to ventilate
6. If previous measures are unsuccessful and equipment is available under an approved protocol, consider advanced airway interventions:
    a. Supraglottic devices
    b. Oro/nasotracheal intubation
    c. Surgical cricothyrotomy
7. Consider applying oxygen if available.

Recovery Position

Unconscious patients should be placed in the semiprone recovery position to prevent the aspiration of blood, mucus, or vomit (**Figure 10-4**). When positioning the patient on his or her side, stabilize the patient's head and move the entire body in a fluid motion. The recovery position counteracts the potential airway obstruction due to spine flexion.

Cricothyrotomy

Emergency cricothyrotomy is a surgical procedure where an incision is made through the skin and cricothyroid membrane. This allows for the placement of a tracheal tube into the trachea when control of the airway is not possible by other methods (**Figure 10-5**).

This procedure has been reported to be safe and effective in trauma victim care. For advanced life support (ALS)-credentialed TECC caregivers working in the indirect threat/warm zone, surgical cricothyrotomy may be appropriate to consider as the next step when a nasopharyngeal airway is not effective assuming they are credentialed within their organization and licensed within their state to do so. It may be the only feasible alternative in cases of maxillofacial wounds in which blood or disrupted anatomy precludes visualization of the vocal cords and the sit-up/lean forward procedure is ineffective in maintaining a secure airway.

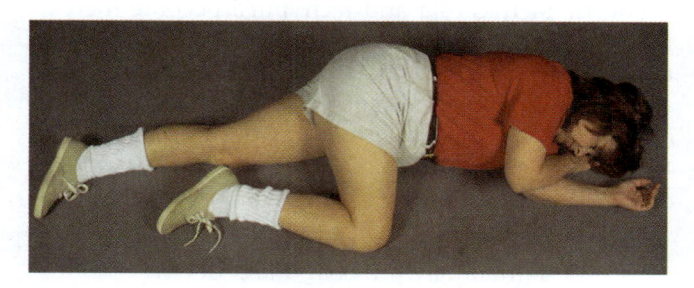

Figure 10-4 Recovery position.
© Jones & Bartlett Learning. Courtesy of MIEMSS.

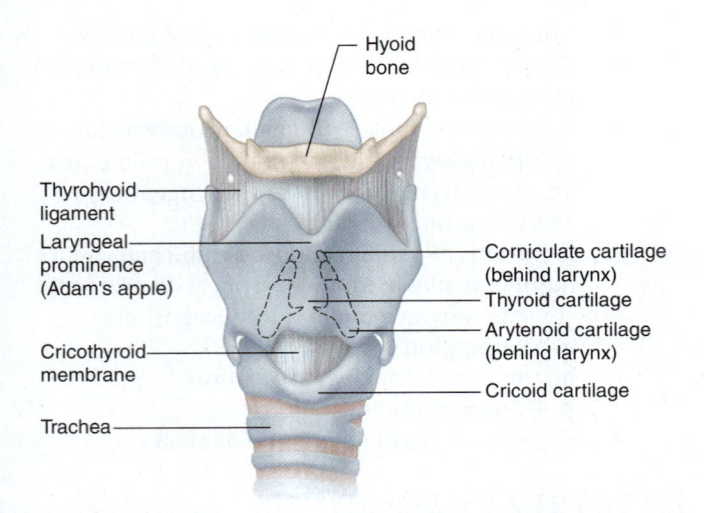

Figure 10-5 Structures involved in a cricothyrotomy.
© Jones & Bartlett Learning. Courtesy of MIEMSS.

CHECK YOUR KNOWLEDGE

Placing the casualty in a recovery position:

a. improves the body's ability to regulate blood pressure.
b. controls brain hemorrhage.
c. identifies which casualties are ready to be evacuated.
d. counteracts the potential airway obstruction due to spine flexion.

Tension Pneumothorax

Tension pneumothorax is the second leading cause of death in the tactical setting. Casualties who remain conscious will generally complain of chest pain and difficulty breathing. As the tension pneumothorax worsens, they will exhibit increasing agitation, tachypnea, and respiratory distress. In severe cases, cyanosis and cardiac arrest may occur.

Physical findings that may be evident are jugular venous distension, absent breath sounds, tracheal deviation away from site of injury, chest wall crepitus, and cyanosis. Tachycardia and tachypnea become increasingly prominent as the intrathoracic pressure builds and the pulse pressure narrows, culminating in hypotension and uncompensated shock.

The priority in management involves decompressing the tension pneumothorax. Decompression should be performed when the following three findings are present:

1. Worsening respiratory distress or difficulty ventilating with a bag-mask device
2. Unilateral decreased or absent breath sounds
3. Decompensated shock (systolic blood pressure <90 mm Hg with a narrowed pulse pressure)

BOX 10-1
Signs of Tension Pneumothorax

Although the following signs are frequently discussed with a tension pneumothorax, many may not be present or are difficult to identify in the field.

Observation
- *Cyanosis* may be difficult to see in the field. Poor lighting, variation in skin color, and dirt and blood associated with trauma often render this sign unreliable.
- *Distended neck veins* are described as a classic sign of tension pneumothorax. However, because a patient with a tension pneumothorax may also have lost a considerable amount of blood, distended neck veins may not be prominent.

Palpation
- *Subcutaneous emphysema* is a common finding. As the pressure builds up within the chest cavity, air will begin to dissect through the tissues of the chest wall. Because tension pneumothorax involves significantly elevated intrathoracic pressure, the subcutaneous emphysema can often be palpated across the entire chest wall and neck and sometimes can involve the abdominal wall and face.
- *Tracheal deviation* is usually a late sign. Even when it is present, it can be difficult to diagnose by physical examination. In the neck, the trachea is bound to the cervical spine by fascial and other supporting structures; thus, the deviation of the trachea is more of an intrathoracic phenomenon, although deviation may be palpated in the jugular notch if it is severe. Tracheal deviation is not often noted in the prehospital environment.

Auscultation
- *Decreased breath sounds on the injured side*. The most helpful part of the physical examination is checking for decreased breath sounds on the side of the injury. However, to use this sign, the prehospital care provider must be able to distinguish between normal and decreased sounds. Such differentiation requires a great deal of practice. Listening to breath sounds during every patient contact will help.

> **CHECK YOUR KNOWLEDGE**
>
> **One sign of tension pneumothorax is:**
>
> a. tracheal deviation toward the side of injury.
> b. flat and flaccid jugular veins.
> c. distended jugular veins.
> d. pulse rate below 60 beats/minute.

Open Pneumothorax

An open pneumothorax involves air entering the pleural space, causing the lung to collapse. When the patient attempts to inhale, air crosses the open wound and enters the pleural space because of the negative pressure created in the thoracic cavity as the muscles of respiration contract. In larger wounds, there may be free flow of air in and out of the pleural space with the different phases of respiration. Audible noise is often created as air travels in and out of the hole in the chest wall; thus, this type of wound has been referred to as a "sucking chest wound" (**Figure 10-6**).

Prehospital Trauma Life Support (PHTLS) recommends the following approach to the management of an open pneumothorax:

1. Place a vented chest seal over the open chest wound.
2. If a vented seal is not available, place a plastic or foil square over the wound and tape on three sides.
3. If none of these is available, an unvented chest seal or a material such as petroleum gauze that prevents ingress and egress of air may be used; however, this approach may allow the development of a tension pneumothorax, so the patient must be observed carefully for signs of deterioration.
4. If the patient develops tachycardia, tachypnea, or other indications of respiratory distress, remove the dressing for a few seconds and assist ventilations as necessary.
5. If respiratory distress continues, assume the development of a tension pneumothorax and perform a needle thoracostomy using a large-bore (10- to 14-gauge) intravenous (IV) needle that is at least 8 cm (3.5 inches) in length. Insert the needle in the fifth intercostal space along the anterior axillary line. Alternatively, insert the needle at the midclavicular line in the second intercostal space.

Most chest wounds do not need to be packed with a gauze dressing. Use a hemostatic dressing and direct pressure.

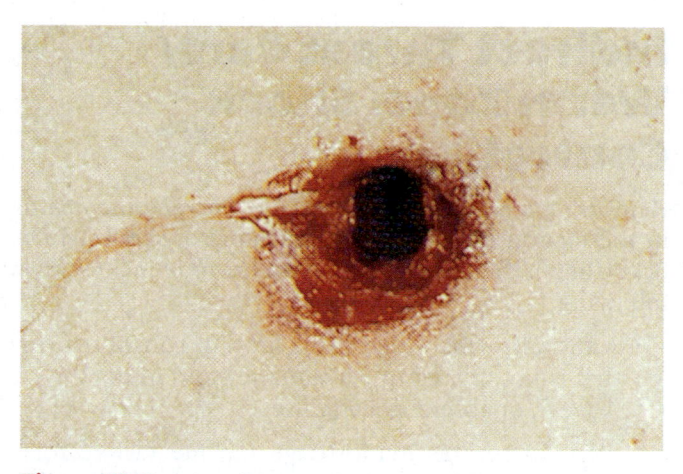

Figure 10-6 A gunshot or stab wound to the chest produces a hole in the chest wall through which air can flow both into and out of the pleural cavity.
Courtesy of Norman McSwain, MD, FACS, NREMT-P.

> **BOX 10-2**
>
> **Should I Take the Dressing Off?**
>
> In the patient with an open pneumothorax, if an occluding dressing has been applied, it should be briefly opened or removed. This should allow the tension pneumothorax to decompress through the wound with a rush of air. This procedure may need to be repeated periodically during transport if symptoms of tension pneumothorax reoccur. If removing the dressing for several seconds is ineffective or if there is no open wound, an ALS provider may proceed with a needle thoracostomy.

> **CHECK YOUR KNOWLEDGE**
>
> **An open chest wound is treated with a foil square that is taped on three sides. The patient is having increased difficulty in breathing with a rapid rise in heart rate. The TECC caregiver should remove the foil and:**
>
> a. pack the wound with gauze.
> b. assist ventilations as needed.
> c. insert advanced airway.
> d. digitally explore the wound for shrapnel.

Indirect Threat Care/Warm Zone: Shock Control

Hemorrhage is the leading cause of preventable death in the tactical environment. Indicators of shock while operating in the indirect threat/warm zone include the following:

- A casualty with a decreased level of consciousness that is not related to a traumatic brain injury
- A weak or absent radial pulse

Signs of serious hemorrhage include tachycardia greater than 120 beats/minute, tachypnea of 30 to 40 breaths/minute, and profound confusion or anxiety. The pulse rate and respiration rate will continue to climb, while the systolic blood pressure will fall to 60 mm Hg. These patients have minutes to live.

TECC caregivers must take measures to control external blood loss, titrate IV electrolyte solution (plasma when available) to a systolic blood pressure of greater than 80 mm Hg, and transport rapidly to the hospital, where blood, plasma, and clotting factors are available and emergent operative steps to control blood loss can be performed, as necessary. The goal is to only provide enough fluid to maintain perfusion and continue to provide oxygenated red blood cells (RBCs) to the heart, brain, and lungs.

> **CHECK YOUR KNOWLEDGE**
>
> **The goal in fluid resuscitation of hemorrhagic shock is to:**
>
> a. aggressively administer crystalloid solutions to get systolic blood pressure to 120 mm Hg.
> b. alternate between crystalloid and plasma administrations to avoid cavitation.
> c. alternate between Ringer lactate and saline to smooth out electrolyte imbalance.
> d. provide just enough fluid to maintain perfusion and continue to provide oxygenated RBCs to the heart, brain, and lungs.

Indirect Threat Care/Warm Zone: Analgesics

The TECC caregiver who is authorized to administer analgesics has a variety of options. For mild to moderate pain, consider oral nonnarcotic medications such as acetaminophen (Tylenol). Avoid the use of nonsteroidal anti-inflammatory (NSAID) medications (e.g., aspirin, ibuprofen, naproxen, ketorolac, etc.) in the trauma patient as these medications interfere with platelet functioning and may exacerbate bleeding.

For severe pain, consider the use of narcotic medications (hydrocodone, oxycodone, transmucosal fentanyl citrate, etc.) as well as ketamine at analgesic dosages. For all opiate administrations have naloxone readily available. Monitor the patient for adverse effects such as respiratory depression or hypotension. Consider adjunct administration of antiemetic medicines. Do not administer narcotic analgesics or ketamine to a responder who remains armed or who must potentially defend him- or herself.

Working in the dynamic indirect threat/warm zone, consider the effect of opioid-induced altered mental status on subsequent operations and required resources. It may be prudent to wait until the patient arrives at the evacuation/cold zone before administering opioids.

> **CHECK YOUR KNOWLEDGE**
>
> **TECC choices for analgesics include all of the following except:**
>
> a. acetaminophen.
> b. ketamine.
> c. aspirin.
> d. oxycodone.

Evacuation Care/Cold Zone

Preparing to move the casualty from the evacuation care/cold zone is similar to moving a trauma patient outside of the tactical arena to a medical facility. TECC caregivers will perform a head-to-toe reassessment of the casualty, checking for bleeding, airway patency, and any life threats. All splints, bandages, and IV lines are reassessed. For casualties who are hemodynamically unstable, these activities will be conducted en route to the hospital if possible based on availability of transport. Never delay transport in an unstable patient for nonlifesaving interventions.

There are two levels of documentation. One is directly on the patient for significant treatment or condition that needs to be conveyed to the receiving facility independent of paper, voice, or electronic notifications. Placement of a tourniquet and establishment of an IV line are two time-sensitive activities that need to be recorded on the patient.

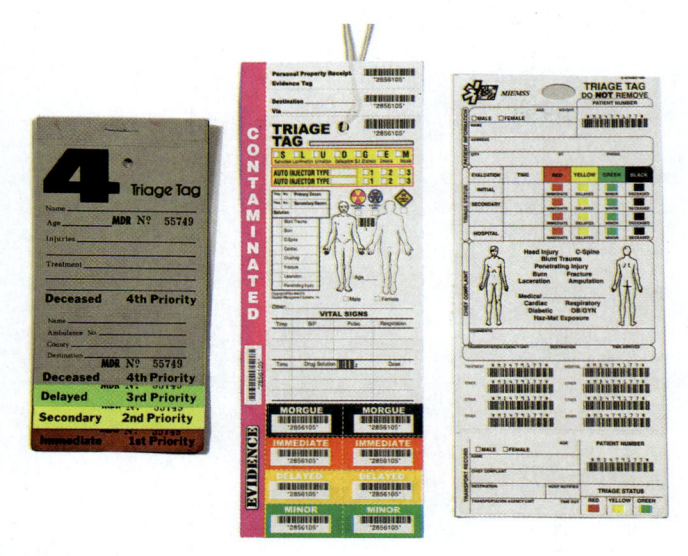

Figure 10-7 Triage tag.
© File of Life Foundation, Inc.

> **CHECK YOUR KNOWLEDGE**
>
> Time-sensitive prehospital treatments that need to be recorded on the patient include:
>
> a. when tourniquet was applied.
> b. size of IV cannula.
> c. initial vital signs.
> d. when rewarming efforts began.

The second level of documentation is the data found on a prehospital care report. Initial observation, prehospital care delivered, vital signs, and patient history are included in the prehospital care report. Due to the austere nature of tactical arenas, this documentation may be found on a triage tag (**Figure 10-7**).

Summary

- Tactical situations present unique challenges as providers attempt to triage patients.
- In addition to sorting casualties, lifesaving interventions should be applied per the MARCH algorithm.
- Algorithmic sorting of casualties is a good baseline but not a substitute for provider intuition and experience.

REFERENCE AND RESOURCE

National Association of Emergency Medical Technicians. *PHTLS: Prehospital Trauma Life Support*. 9th ed. Burlington, MA: Public Safety Group; 2019.

Answers to Check Your Knowledge

Lesson 1: Introduction to Tactical Emergency Casualty Care

CHECK YOUR KNOWLEDGE

TECC guidelines cover the medical requirements of:

a. fit and healthy 18- to 40-year-old first responders.
b. emergency medical services responders.
c. those most likely to survive a multisystem trauma injury.
d. the civilian population.

Answer: D. the civilian population.

Rationale: TECC guidelines cover the requirements of a civilian population.

CHECK YOUR KNOWLEDGE

You have successfully completed the TECC course and are operating in an indirect threat care/warm zone scene. Your patient has a tension pneumothorax, is rapidly decompensating, and needs a needle decompression. You can perform this skill under which of these situations?

a. On-site medical oversight is available by a critical care paramedic or physician assistant.
b. The caregiver calls medical control, identifies as a TECC-credentialed caregiver, and obtains authorization.
c. Needle decompression is within the caregiver's scope of practice and authorized under local policy and protocol.
d. The incident has been declared a mass-casualty event and the authority having jurisdiction has established medical incident command under the National Response Framework.

Answer: C. Needle decompression is within the caregiver's scope of practice and authorized under local policy and protocol.

Rationale: Outside of class, all clinical interventions must be in accordance with local policy and protocol and within the caregiver's authorized scope of practice.

CHECK YOUR KNOWLEDGE

The use of advanced airway devices can start in the _____ zone.

a. direct threat/hot
b. indirect threat/warm
c. evacuation/cold
d. All of the zones

Answer: B. indirect threat/warm

Rationale: Warm zone care includes the other lifesaving interventions associated with applying the MARCH algorithm.

CHECK YOUR KNOWLEDGE

When operating in a tactical situation _____ can sometimes be _____ and cause mission failure.

a. response teams; attacked
b. too many paramedics; uncoordinated
c. good medicine; bad tactics
d. EMT-level caregivers; overwhelmed

Answer: C. good medicine; bad tactics

Rationale: Good medicine can sometimes be bad tactics, and bad tactics can get everyone killed and/or cause mission failure.

CHECK YOUR KNOWLEDGE

_____ focuses on medical care of the first responders.

a. Medical branch
b. Tactical emergency medical support
c. Rescue task force
d. Police medic

Answer: B. Tactical emergency medical support

Rationale: This differs from rescue task force, which usually focuses on medical care for tactical casualties.

Lesson 2: Direct Threat Care/Hot Zone

CHECK YOUR KNOWLEDGE

The zone that represents the highest danger to caregiver and patient is the _____ zone.

a. tactical
b. direct threat
c. indirect threat
d. evacuation care

Answer: B. direct threat

Rationale: The direct threat zone represents the highest danger to caregiver and patient.

CHECK YOUR KNOWLEDGE

Which is a key factor of remote assessment methodology?

a. The caregiver is embedded with the casualty until the direct threat is mitigated.
b. The caregiver is unable to get direction from online medical control.
c. The caregiver is unable to touch the patient.
d. Sending live video from the direct threat/hot zone to the medical sector

Answer: C. The caregiver is unable to touch the patient.

Rationale: Remote medical assessment is the process of assessing and rendering aid to those who are out of direct physical and visual contact of the provider.

CHECK YOUR KNOWLEDGE

What is the quickest medical intervention while operating in direct threat/hot zone?

a. Hemorrhage control
b. Rapid extrication
c. Passive airway maintenance
d. Tactical hypotension

Answer: C. Passive airway maintenance

Rationale: A TECC caregiver may only have the time to place the patient in the recovery position.

Lesson 3: Indirect Threat Care/Warm Zone: MARCH—Patient Assessment and Massive Hemorrhage Interventions

CHECK YOUR KNOWLEDGE

Deploying a fire company hose line to obscure or interfere with an active shooter's line-of-sight is an example of:

a. freelancing.
b. responding with overwhelming response.
c. asymmetric response.
d. fortifying the rescue corridor.

Answer: C. asymmetric response.

Rationale: Direct threats should receive asymmetric rescue responses.

CHECK YOUR KNOWLEDGE

What does "raking" during a blood sweep mean?

a. Removing all clothing during assessment
b. Spreading the fingers of your gloved hands and using your fingers to palpate the patient
c. Making your gloved hand into a fist and using your knuckles to palpate the patient
d. Placing the fingers of your gloved hand into a "V" and vigorously tapping on the patient

Answer: B. Spreading the fingers of your gloved hand and using your fingers to palpate the patient

Rationale: Raking means assessing by spreading your fingers out and curving them in, resembling a rake you would you use to remove leaves from a lawn.

CHECK YOUR KNOWLEDGE

When using PACE methodology in hemorrhagic control, wound packing would be an example of which step?

a. Primary
b. Alternative
c. Contingency
d. Emergency

Answer: C. Contingency

Rationale: Contingency: Wound packing, junctional tourniquet.

CHECK YOUR KNOWLEDGE

When is tourniquet conversion indicated?

a. Evacuation to hospital-level care is more than 2 hours.
b. Patient exhibits signs of traumatic brain injury.
c. Patient is hypotensive.
d. Limb has swollen.

Answer: A. Evacuation to hospital-level care is more than 2 hours.

Rationale: Tourniquet conversion may be indicated if evacuation to hospital-level definitive care is significantly more than 2 hours.

CHECK YOUR KNOWLEDGE

After packing Combat Gauze into a wound and applying pressure until the bleeding stops, you need to hold continuous pressure for at least _____ minutes.

a. 15
b. 10
c. 8
d. 3

Answer: D. 3

Rationale: Hold continuous pressure for at least 3 minutes per manufacturer guidelines.

Lesson 4: Indirect Threat Care/Warm Zone: MARCH—Airway

CHECK YOUR KNOWLEDGE

Which of these is the easiest and most effective technique to maintain an airway for an unresponsive patient under tactical conditions?

a. Surgical airway
b. Endotracheal intubation
c. Oropharyngeal airway
d. Nasopharyngeal airway

Answer: D. Nasopharyngeal airway

Rationale: If spontaneous respirations are present and there is no respiratory distress, an adequate airway may be maintained in an unconscious or unresponsive patient by the insertion of a nasopharyngeal airway.

CHECK YOUR KNOWLEDGE

A bag-mask device is required when using a(n) _____ to maintain an airway.

a. oropharyngeal airway
b. supraglottic airway
c. nasopharyngeal airway
d. esophageal shunt

Answer: B. supraglottic airway

Rationale: In addition to the supraglottic airway, the casualty may need to be ventilated using a bag-mask device or ventilator.

CHECK YOUR KNOWLEDGE

A cricothyrotomy incision is made to the:

a. cricoid cartilage.
b. thyroid cartilage.
c. cricothyroid membrane.
d. thyroid prominence.

Answer: C. cricothyroid membrane.

Rationale: A cricothyrotomy is the surgical placement of a hole in the cricothyroid membrane.

CHECK YOUR KNOWLEDGE

Which of these is an important anatomic difference to consider with airway control in a pediatric patient?

a. Larger tongue
b. Lower tidal volume
c. Reduced size discrepancy between the cranium and midface
d. Posterior positioned airway

Answer: A. Larger tongue

Rationale: Children have a relatively large occiput and tongue and have an anteriorly positioned airway.

Lesson 5: Indirect Threat Care/Warm Zone: Respiration/Breathing

CHECK YOUR KNOWLEDGE

Generating negative pressure during inspiration requires a(n):

a. intact chest wall.
b. adequate cardiac output.
c. systolic blood pressure above 50 mm Hg.
d. intact alveoli structure.

Answer: A. intact chest wall.

Rationale: Generating negative pressure during inspiration requires an intact chest wall.

CHECK YOUR KNOWLEDGE

A casualty with an open pneumothorax always:

a. requires spinal immobilization.
b. presents with distended neck veins.
c. requires evaluation for cardiac tamponade.
d. has an injury to the underlying lung.

Answer: D. has an injury to the underlying lung.

Rationale: A patient with an open pneumothorax virtually always has an injury to the underlying lung.

CHECK YOUR KNOWLEDGE

Which is a late sign with tension pneumothorax?

a. anxiety
b. diminished/absent breath sounds
c. tracheal deviation
d. unequal chest rise and fall

Answer: C. Tracheal deviation

Rationale: Tracheal deviation is a rare and very late finding of tension pneumothorax. It is not typically encountered in the prehospital setting. Anxiety, diminished/absent breath sounds, and unequal chest rise and fall (answers A, B, and D) are all earlier signs of tension pneumothorax.

CHECK YOUR KNOWLEDGE

A needle/catheter size appropriate for decompression is _____ gauge

a. 8
b. 14
c. 18
d. 22

Answer: B. 14

Rationale: Regardless of the method chosen, decompression should be performed with a large-bore (10- to 16-gauge) IV needle that is at least 8 cm (3.5 inches) in length.

Lesson 6: Indirect Threat Care/Warm Zone: MARCH—Circulation

CHECK YOUR KNOWLEDGE

Insufficient tourniquet compression will:

a. increase the rate of sepsis in the damaged limb.
b. generate circulatory embolisms.
c. cause loss of blood to the general circulation.
d. postpone the onset of shock.

Answer: C. cause loss of blood to the general circulation.

Rationale: The trapped blood causes limb edema and loss of blood to the general circulation, which can hasten the onset of shock.

CHECK YOUR KNOWLEDGE

Shock is defined as:

a. pulse rate at more than 140 beats per minute.
b. inadequate tissue perfusion at the cellular level.
c. diastolic blood pressure of less than 50 mm Hg for more than 20 minutes.
d. pulse-oximeter SpO_2 reading of less than 84%.

Answer: B. inadequate tissue perfusion at the cellular level.

Rationale: The correct definition of shock is inadequate tissue perfusion (oxygenation) at the cellular level that leads to anaerobic metabolism and insufficient energy production needed to support life. Pulse rate, blood pressure, and pulse oximetry may be normal in patients despite the presence of shock.

CHECK YOUR KNOWLEDGE

How is the transition from compensated to decompensated hypovolemic shock identified?

a. Blood pressure drops.
b. Pulse rate drops below 50 beats per minute.
c. Patient starts to sweat copiously.
d. Patient starts a run of vigorous, unproductive coughing.

Answer: A. Blood pressure drops.

Rationale: This decrease in blood pressure marks the switch from compensated to decompensated shock—a sign of impending death. Pulse rate is typically high in these patients. Sweating copiously begins with uncompensated shock. Coughing is not typically associated with this transition.

CHECK YOUR KNOWLEDGE

The sympathetic nervous system is capable of handling a Class _____ hemorrhage situation.

a. II
b. III
c. IV
d. The sympathetic nervous system is incapable of handling a hemorrhage situation.

Answer: A. II

Rationale: Most adults are capable of compensating for this amount of blood loss by activation of the sympathetic nervous system, which will maintain their blood pressure. Class III hemorrhage is typically associated with the onset of decompensated shock, which means that the sympathetic nervous system is no longer capable of compensating for the volume of blood that has been lost from the circulation.

CHECK YOUR KNOWLEDGE

Narrow pulse pressure distinguishes _____ shock from _____ shock.

a. hemorrhagic; pulmonary
b. hypovolemic; neurogenic
c. neurogenic; cardiogenic
d. neurogenic; pulmonary

Answer: B. hypovolemic; neurogenic

Rationale: Decreased systolic and diastolic pressures and a narrow pulse pressure characterize hypovolemic shock. These findings are typically not associated with neurogenic shock or cardiogenic shock. There is no specific entity named pulmonary shock.

CHECK YOUR KNOWLEDGE

You are treating a patient in the indirect threat care/warm zone who has a gunshot wound to the gut and a systolic blood pressure of 90 by palpation. There will be a 15- to 20-minute delay in moving the patient to the evacuation care/cold zone. What is the most appropriate fluid resuscitation?

a. No fluid resuscitation in the indirect threat care/warm zone
b. 18-gauge needle with saline lock
c. Intraosseous access and one IV line of a crystalloid solution
d. Two 14-guage IV lines flowing lactated Ringer

Answer: B. 18-gauge needle with saline lock

Rationale: One 18-gauge needle with saline lock is the correct answer. Fluid resuscitation should be withheld as long as the casualty's blood pressure remains above 80 mm Hg. Two 14-gauge IV lines (answer D) is an old technique associated with older resuscitation protocols that involved massive crystalloid infusions. These are now recognized to be associated with increased rates of pulmonary complications and increased bleeding due to dilution of clotting factors and excessive blood pressure in the context of ongoing hemorrhage. While this patient does not need resuscitation now (answer A), answer B is preferable since his or her condition could easily deteriorate further and blood pressure could fall below 90 mm Hg to 80 mm Hg or less, in which case urgent fluid administration would be desirable.

CHECK YOUR KNOWLEDGE

What is the goal in fluid resuscitation of hemorrhagic shock?

a. Aggressively administer crystalloid solutions to get systolic blood pressure to 120 mm Hg.
b. Alternate between crystalloid and plasma administrations to avoid cavitation.
c. Alternate between Ringer lactate and saline to smooth out electrolyte imbalance.
d. Provide just enough fluid to maintain perfusion and continue to provide oxygenated RBCs to the heart, brain, and lungs.

Answer: D. Provide just enough fluid to maintain perfusion and continue to provide oxygenated RBCs to the heart, brain, and lungs.

Rationale: Provide only enough fluid to maintain perfusion and continue to provide oxygenated RBCs to the heart, brain, and lungs. This allows for maintenance of viability until hemorrhage can be definitively controlled and resuscitation with blood can be initiated.

CHECK YOUR KNOWLEDGE

You are administering an IV dose of TXA and the patient complains of dizziness and vomits. You should:

a. speed up the rate of TXA infusion.
b. slow down the rate of TXA infusion.
c. stop IV administration of TXA.
d. check patient blood pressure, and stop TXA if systolic is below 60 mm Hg.

Answer: B. slow down the rate of TXA infusion.

Rationale: If there is a new-onset drop in blood pressure during the infusion, *slow down* the TXA infusion.

CHECK YOUR KNOWLEDGE

A casualty with signs of traumatic brain injury and hypotension:

a. is triaged as a gray/black tag patient.
b. requires fluid resuscitation to maintain a normal radial pulse.
c. must be hyperventilated with high-flow oxygen.
d. needs to be transported in the Trendelenburg position.

Answer: B. requires fluid resuscitation to maintain a normal radial pulse.

Rationale: Patients with a suspected traumatic brain injury who also present with a weak or absent pulse need fluid resuscitation. The goal is to restore a normal radial pulse. Black triage tags are reserved for obviously dead patients or patients who are expected to expire. Hyperventilation is contraindicated for these patients unless there is active evidence of herniation. Trendelenberg should generally be avoided for these patients in order to decrease intracranial pressure. Reverse Trendelenberg may be valuable if blood pressure can be maintained.

Lesson 7: Indirect Threat Care/Warm Zone: Hypothermia and Head Injury

CHECK YOUR KNOWLEDGE

A moderate traumatic brain injury would have a Glasgow Coma Scale score of:

a. 13 to 15.
b. 9 to 12.
c. 3 to 8.
d. 0 to 3.

Answer: B. 9 to 12.

Rationale: A GCS score of 9 to 12 is indicative of moderate TBI.

CHECK YOUR KNOWLEDGE

The initial blood pressure is taken:

a. on arrival to the indirect threat care/warm zone.
b. during the secondary survey.
c. just prior to leaving the indirect threat care/warm zone.
d. just prior to leaving the evacuation care/cold zone.

Answer: B. during the secondary survey.

Rationale: The secondary survey is the point during the indirect threat care/warm zone where the TECC provider obtains and records vital signs.

CHECK YOUR KNOWLEDGE

TECC choices for analgesics include all of the following, *except*:

a. acetaminophen.
b. ketamine.
c. aspirin.
d. oxycodone.

Answer: C. aspirin.

Rationale: Avoid the use of nonsteroidal anti-inflammatory (NSAID) medications (e.g., aspirin, ibuprofen, naproxen, ketorolac, etc.).

Answers to Check Your Knowledge

CHECK YOUR KNOWLEDGE

Which is an issue with a fire-based terror attack?

a. Intense smoke
b. Threat of explosives
c. Low-to-no visibility
d. All of these are correct.

Answer: D. All of these are correct.

Rationale: The scene may include fire, intense smoke, low-to-no visibility, and the threat of firearms and explosives.

CHECK YOUR KNOWLEDGE

A secondary survey reveals a small piece of shrapnel imbedded in the patient's eye. TECC guidelines call for the caregiver to:

a. initiate a 20-minute flush with saline solution.
b. prepare and place a doughnut ring around the shrapnel.
c. tape a rigid eye shield over the injured eye.
d. cover both eyes with occlusive dressing.

Answer: C. tape a rigid eye shield over the injured eye.

Rationale: TECC guidelines recommend the use of a rigid eye shield without padding. The objective is to provide a hard barrier between the impaled eye and the environment. Any padding under the rigid shield may stick to the eye or increase intraocular pressure.

CHECK YOUR KNOWLEDGE

When preparing to move casualties from the indirect threat care/warm zone to the evacuation care/cold zone:

a. wait for the appropriate number of ambulance teams to arrive at the warm zone/cold zone border.
b. coordinate with the incident management team.
c. determine the smoothest path with the fewest obstacles.
d. take the same path you used to get to the indirect threat care/warm zone.

Answer: B. coordinate with the incident management team.

Rationale: This requires coordination with the incident management team and the security status of the hot zone threats.

CHECK YOUR KNOWLEDGE

While triaging patients in the indirect threat care/warm zone you encounter a casualty with multiple system trauma who has no pulse. The TECC recommendation is to:

a. triage patient as gray or black tag.
b. perform the head tilt maneuver to see if respiration returns.
c. do three cycles of continuous closed chest compressions, and then check for a pulse.
d. perform bilateral needle chest decompressions, and then check for a pulse.

Answer: D. perform bilateral needle chest decompressions, and then check for a pulse.

Rationale: TECC guidelines have the caregiver consider bilateral needle decompression for nonbreathing and pulseless casualties with torso or polytrauma (two or more significant trauma injuries).

Lesson 8: Evacuation Care/Cold Zone

CHECK YOUR KNOWLEDGE

Evacuation care means medical care:

a. delivered upon arrival to a hospital or medical center.
b. provided during transport from the cold zone to the hospital or medical center.
c. provided while the casualty is in the cold zone.
d. provided during the movement of the casualty from the warm zone to the cold zone.

Answer: C. provided while the casualty is in the cold zone.

Rationale: For TECC providers this is evacuation care—the kind of casualty care provided by TECC caregivers after rescuing casualties from a dangerous place.

CHECK YOUR KNOWLEDGE

A significant difference in evacuation care/cold zone is:

a. better ventilation and lighting.
b. more caregivers and resources available.
c. ability to interact with the incident commander.
d. tighter security.

Answer: B. more caregivers and resources available.

Rationale: At evacuation/cold zone care there are more caregivers and resources available.

CHECK YOUR KNOWLEDGE

The primary advantage of using a supraglottic airway is that it:

a. provides positive control of the trachea.
b. completely eliminates the risk of aspiration.
c. introduces high concentrations of oxygen.
d. may be inserted independent of the patient's position.

Answer: D. may be inserted independent of the patient's position.

Rationale: A supraglottic airway may be inserted independent of the patient's position. The disadvantage is that it provides incomplete control of the trachea in that it only partially protects it from gastric contents and aspiration in the event of vomiting. All available airway devices can be used to introduce high-flow oxygen.

CHECK YOUR KNOWLEDGE

A needle decompression requires an IV needle of _____ gauge or larger.

a. 22
b. 20
c. 18
d. 16

Answer: D. 16

Rationale: Decompression should be performed with a large-bore (10- to 16-gauge) IV needle that is at least 8 cm (3.5 inches) in length.

CHECK YOUR KNOWLEDGE

Assessing the casualty for hemorrhage includes:

a. loosening tourniquets applied in the hot zone.
b. performing the rake procedure.
c. palpating systolic blood pressure.
d. blanching fingernails.

Answer: B. performing the rake procedure.

Rationale: A combination of raking and sweeping is more effective. Tourniquets should not be removed once applied unless they are too loose. Palpating the systolic blood pressure is also a measure of potential hemorrhage, but less specific than identifying it visually. Blanching fingernails and assessing for capillary refill is primarily useful to assess perfusion in children.

CHECK YOUR KNOWLEDGE

Which is a contraindication for tourniquet conversion?

a. Utilization of the pelvic binder
b. Lack of hemostatic agent
c. Patient has received colloids or whole blood.
d. Transport time to the hospital is anticipated to be 90 minutes.

Answer: D. Transport time to the hospital is anticipated to be 90 minutes.

Rationale: Conversion should not be attempted unless total tourniquet time is expected to substantially exceed 2 hours.

CHECK YOUR KNOWLEDGE

The goal of evacuation care/cold zone fluid resuscitation for patients without traumatic brain injury is to:

a. maintain a systolic blood pressure between 120 and 130 mm Hg.
b. maintain a diastolic blood pressure between 80 and 90 mm Hg.
c. increase the number of red blood cells.
d. maintain a palpable radial pulse.

Answer: D. maintain a palpable radial pulse.

Rationale: Administration of lactated Ringer or normal saline should continue until systolic blood pressure is above 80 mm Hg.

CHECK YOUR KNOWLEDGE

_____ more than doubles the risk of death from brain injury.

a. Uneven pupillary response to light
b. Decorticate posturing
c. Systolic blood pressure >120 mm Hg
d. Oxygen saturation via pulse oximetry (SpO_2) <90%

Answer: D. Oxygen saturation via pulse oximetry (SpO_2) <90%

Rationale: Oxygen saturation via pulse oximetry (SpO_2) <90% more than doubles the risk of death from brain injury.

CHECK YOUR KNOWLEDGE

Which of these statements regarding smoke inhalation patients is true?

a. Do not intubate a soot-soaked trachea.
b. Hydroxocobalamin may be a better antidote for cyanide poisoning.
c. Sodium thiosulfate is the first IV medication to use in cyanide poisoning situations.
d. The pulse oximetry device doubles the SpO_2 value in instances of carbon monoxide poisoning.

Answer: B. Hydroxocobalamin may be a better antidote for cyanide poisoning.

Rationale: Hydroxocobalamin, which was approved by the Food and Drug Administration in 2006, has a more positive risk–benefit profile and may be a better antidote for cyanide poisoning.

CHECK YOUR KNOWLEDGE

A cause for a traumatic cardiac arrest in the evacuation care/cold zone could be:

a. exsanguination.
a. herniated brain.
b. airway compromise.
c. All of these are correct.

Answer: D. All of these are correct.

Rationale: The TECC caregiver should consider the underlying clinical cause for the cardiac arrest, which may include exsanguination, herniated brain, or airway compromise.

CHECK YOUR KNOWLEDGE

The presence of hypothermia and acidosis can result in _____ mortality in severe trauma patients.

a. 90%
b. 70%
c. 60%
d. 40%

Answer: A. 90%

Rationale: The presence of hypothermia and acidosis, which results in coagulopathy, and the relationship among these three conditions, can result in a 90% death rate among victims of severe trauma.

CHECK YOUR KNOWLEDGE

Time-sensitive prehospital treatments that need to be recorded on the patient include:

a. when tourniquet was applied.
b. size of IV cannula.
c. initial vital signs.
d. when rewarming efforts began.

Answer: A. when tourniquet was applied.

Rationale: Placement of a tourniquet and establishment of an IV line are two time-sensitive activities that need to be recorded on the patient.

Lesson 9: Triage

CHECK YOUR KNOWLEDGE

A casualty triaged as _____ may be engaged as a patient mover.

a. immediate
b. delayed
c. minor
d. expectant

Answer: C. minor.

Rationale: A minor casualty may even assist in the interim by comforting other patients or helping as litter bearers.

CHECK YOUR KNOWLEDGE

A main activity in primary triage is to:

a. document baseline vital signs on each patient.
b. document the triage classification on each patient.
c. determine the number of guns and caliber of weapons in use.
d. determine the level of chemical exposure.

Answer: B. document the triage classification on each patient.

Rationale: During primary triage, patients are briefly assessed and then identified in some way, usually by attaching a triage tag or triage tape.

CHECK YOUR KNOWLEDGE

A critique of triage systems:

a. focuses on identifying individuals needing a trauma center.
b. identifies the number of casualties and level of priority.
c. provides a scope of the incident to the incident commander.
d. provides earliest notice of transport requirements.

Answer: A. focuses on identifying individuals needing a trauma center.

Rationale: In-field triage is intended to allow prehospital personnel to determine whether a single given patient requires the resources of a trauma center.

CHECK YOUR KNOWLEDGE

A patient who is breathing faster than 30 breaths/min is triaged as:

a. immediate.
b. delayed.
c. Imminent.
d. minor.

Answer: A. immediate.

Rationale: A patient who is breathing faster than 30 breaths/min or slower than 10 breaths/min is triaged as an immediate priority (red).

CHECK YOUR KNOWLEDGE

In what way does the SALT method differ from other triage systems?

a. Utilization of on-line medical control
b. Use of lifesaving steps as part of triage assessment
c. Focusing on patients who can wave but not walk
d. Faster processing of patients to the transport section

Answer: B. Use of lifesaving steps as part of triage assessment

Rationale: The SALT method differs from others in its lifesaving intervention steps, which include bleeding control, opening the airway, two rescue breaths for children, needle decompression for tension pneumothorax, and autoinjector antidotes.

CHECK YOUR KNOWLEDGE

Secondary triage includes analysis of _____ and _____.

a. anticipated tactical situation; patient response to MARCH treatments
b. immediate tactical situation; patient vital signs
c. projected tactical situation; patient vital signs
d. immediate tactical situation; patient response to MARCH treatments

Answer: D. immediate tactical situation; patient response to MARCH treatments

Rationale: The immediate tactical situation and patient response to treatment guide the secondary triage decisions.

Lesson 10: Summation

CHECK YOUR KNOWLEDGE

TECC caregivers' first responsibility is:

a. rapid assessment of patients in direct threat/hot zone.
b. triage of patients in indirect threat/warm zone.
c. scene safety.
d. medical oversight of buddy-care and self-care efforts.

Answer: C. scene safety.

Rationale: TECC caregivers' first responsibility is to ensure scene safety. If caregivers become victims, they can no longer deliver care and they increase the burden of total care that must be delivered by the remaining cadre of responders.

CHECK YOUR KNOWLEDGE

The MARCH algorithm is exercised in the _____ zone.

a. hot
b. transitional
c. warm
d. evacuation

Answer: C. warm

Rationale: Warm zone care includes the other lifesaving interventions associated with applying the MARCH algorithm (**M**assive hemorrhage, **A**irway, **R**espiration, **C**irculation, and **H**ypothermia/**H**ead injury).

CHECK YOUR KNOWLEDGE

The primary medical priority in the direct threat/hot zone is:

a. assure patent airway.
b. complete initial triage.
c. stop compressible hemorrhage.
d. complete RAM assessment.

Answer: C. stop compressible hemorrhage.

Rationale: Compressible severe external hemorrhage can usually be quickly controlled and should be the first priority.

CHECK YOUR KNOWLEDGE

The primary medical priority in the indirect threat/warm zone is:

a. *do not delay* patient extraction/evacuation for nonlifesaving interventions.
b. stage patient extraction/evacuation until the patient is stabilized and documented.
c. develop patient extrication schedule with the operational medical director or command physician.
d. develop transportation schedule with the transportation section.

Answer: A. *do not delay* patient extraction/evacuation for nonlifesaving interventions.

Rationale: The indirect threat/warm zone goals are:

1. Maintain operational control to stabilize the immediate scenario.
2. Conduct dedicated patient assessment and initiate appropriate lifesaving interventions.
3. *Do not delay* patient extraction/evacuation for nonlifesaving interventions.
4. Consider establishing a patient/casualty collection point.

CHECK YOUR KNOWLEDGE

Control of hemorrhage in the groin, buttock, and axilla is accomplished using:

a. junctional tourniquets.
b. tranexamic acid.
c. both junctional tourniquets and tranexamic acid.
d. neither junctional tourniquets nor tranexamic acid.

Answer: C. both junctional tourniquets and tranexamic acid.

Rationale: Junctional tourniquets may help control hemorrhage in the groin, buttocks, perineum, axilla, and base of the neck. Tranexamic acid can be administered intravenously, by mouth, or directly on a wound to decrease transfusion requirements and improve mortality after hemorrhagic shock.

CHECK YOUR KNOWLEDGE

Placing the casualty in a recovery position:

a. improves the body's ability to regulate blood pressure.
b. controls brain hemorrhage.
c. identifies which casualties are ready to be evacuated.
d. counteracts the potential airway obstruction due to spine flexion.

Answer: D. counteracts the potential airway obstruction due to spine flexion.

Rationale: The recovery position counteracts the potential airway obstruction due to spine flexion.

CHECK YOUR KNOWLEDGE

One sign of tension pneumothorax is:

a. tracheal deviation toward the side of injury.
b. flat and flaccid jugular veins.
c. distended jugular veins.
d. pulse rate below 60 beats/minute.

Answer: C. distended jugular veins.

Rationale: Physical findings that may be evident are jugular venous distension, absent breath sounds, tracheal deviation away from site of injury, chest wall crepitus, and cyanosis.

CHECK YOUR KNOWLEDGE

An open chest wound is treated with a foil square that is taped on three sides. The patient is having increased difficulty in breathing with a rapid rise in heart rate. The TECC caregiver should remove the foil and:

a. pack the wound with gauze.
b. assist ventilations as needed.
c. insert advanced airway.
d. digitally explore the wound for shrapnel.

Answer: B. assist ventilations as needed.

Rationale: If the patient develops tachycardia, tachypnea, or other indications of respiratory distress, remove the dressing for a few seconds and assist ventilations as necessary.

CHECK YOUR KNOWLEDGE

The goal in fluid resuscitation of hemorrhagic shock is to:

a. aggressively administer crystalloid solutions to get systolic blood pressure to 120 mm Hg.
b. alternate between crystalloid and plasma administrations to avoid cavitation.
c. alternate between Ringer lactate and saline to smooth out electrolyte imbalance.
d. provide just enough fluid to maintain perfusion and continue to provide oxygenated RBCs to the heart, brain, and lungs.

Answer: D. provide just enough fluid to maintain perfusion and continue to provide oxygenated RBCs to the heart, brain, and lungs.

Rationale: Provide only enough fluid to maintain perfusion and continue to provide oxygenated RBCs to the heart, brain, and lungs. This allows for maintenance of viability until hemorrhage can be definitively controlled and resuscitation with blood can be initiated.

CHECK YOUR KNOWLEDGE

TECC choices for analgesics include all of the following *except*:

a. acetaminophen.
b. ketamine.
c. aspirin.
d. oxycodone.

Answer: C. aspirin.

Rationale: Avoid the use of nonsteroidal anti-inflammatory (NSAID) medications (e.g., aspirin, ibuprofen, naproxen, ketorolac, etc.).

CHECK YOUR KNOWLEDGE

Time-sensitive prehospital treatments that need to be recorded on the patient include:

a. when tourniquet was applied.
b. size of IV cannula.
c. initial vital signs.
d. when rewarming efforts began.

Answer: A. when tourniquet was applied.

Rationale: Placement of a tourniquet and establishment of an IV line are two time-sensitive activities that need to be recorded on the patient.

Index

Note: Page numbers followed by *b*, *f* and *t* denote materials in boxes, figures and tables.

A

acetaminophen (Tylenol), 75, 114, 123, 130
acidosis, 95, 127
active shooter/hostile events (ASHEs), 3, 4
   scene safety, 17
Adam's apple, 32
advanced airway devices, for indirect threat care/warm zone, 3, 117
advanced life support (ALS), 47
air in pleural space. *See* open pneumothorax
airway
   evacuation care/cold zone, 85, 86*f*
   indirect threat care/warm zone. *See* indirect threat care/warm zone, airway in
ALS. *See* advanced life support
altered mental status, 18, 18*f*
   with suspected traumatic brain injury, 91
ambulance bus, 84, 84*f*
amyl nitrite, 92–93
analgesia
   evacuation care/cold zone, 93, 94*f*
   indirect threat care/warm zone, 75, 79, 114
arterial hemorrhage, 12
arterial tourniquets, 55
Asherman chest seal, 45, 45*f*
ASHEs. *See* active shooter/hostile events
asymmetrical response, 18, 18*f*, 118
axillary hemorrhage, 25

B

BACT. *See* bougie-assisted emergency cricothyrotomy technique
bag-mask device, 29–31, 120
BATS. *See* Bomb Arson Tracking System
bilateral needle decompression for traumatic cardiac arrest, 50
bleeding. *See also* hemorrhage control
   assessment, 19, 19*f*
blind nasotracheal intubation (BNTI), 31
blood pressure, during secondary survey, 74, 123
blood sweep-and-rake assessment, 19

BNTI. *See* blind nasotracheal intubation
body recovery, 8
Bomb Arson Tracking System (BATS), 76
bomb threats, 76*f*
bombs as weapon. *See* fire and bombs as weapons
Bone Injection Gun, 62
Boston Marathon bombing, 1*f*, 107*f*
bougie-assisted emergency cricothyrotomy technique (BACT), 35, 35*f*, 36*f*
burn care
   evacuation care/cold zone, 91
      amyl nitrite, 92
      CYANOKIT, 92, 92*f*
      hydrogen cyanide poisoning protocol, 92–93
      sodium thiosulfate, 92
   indirect threat care/warm zone, 76–77
      analgesia, 79
      assessment of burn injury, 77–78, 77*f*, 78*f*
      fluid resuscitation of burned patients, 78, 78*b*
      smoke inhalation, fluid management considerations, 78–79
burn depth, 77
burn injury, assessment of, 77–78, 77*f*, 78*f*

C

carbon dioxide, 42, 42*f*
carbon monoxide poisoning, 92*b*
cardiogenic shock, 57, 57*t*
   signs associated with, 61*t*
cardiopulmonary resuscitation (CPR)
   evacuation care/cold zone, 93–94
   indirect threat care/warm zone, 80
CAT. *See* Combat Application Tourniquet
Celox Gauze, 24
chaotic "fog of response," 18
chest seals, 46–47
   Asherman, 45, 45*f*
   Halo, 45, 45*f*
   SAM, 45, 45*f*
   vented, 46*f*
chest wall
   intact, 41, 44
   proximity of, 46*f*
Cheyne-Stokes respirations, 72
Chitogauze, 24
chitosan, 24

circulation, indirect threat care/warm zone
   damage control resuscitation
      coagulopathy and "lethal triad," 65–66
      TECC damage control resuscitation, 66
   intraosseous access, 62–64, 62*f*, 63–64*f*, 66–67
   intravenous access, 62–64, 62*f*, 63–64*f*
   pelvic binders, 55–56, 56*f*
      application of, 56
      indications and contraindications for use, 56
      pelvic fractures stabilization, 56
      pelvic hemorrhage control, 56
   shock
      assessment, 56–57, 57*t*
      fluid resuscitation of hemorrhagic shock, 60
      hemorrhagic, 58–60, 58*f*, 59*f*, 59*t*, 60*f*
      hypovolemic, 58
      neurogenic, 61–62
      signs associated with types, 61*t*
   tourniquet
      application, 54–55, 55*b*, 54*f*
      application tightness, 55
      assessment, 53–54, 54*f*
      time limit, 55
   tranexamic acid, 64–65
      administration, 65, 67
   traumatic brain injury, 66
civilian population, medical requirements of, 2, 117
Class I hemorrhage, 58, 59*f*
Class II hemorrhage, 58, 59*f*, 122
Class III hemorrhage, 58–59, 59*f*
Class IV hemorrhage, 59–60, 60*f*
Clinical Randomization of an Antifibrinolytic in Significant Hemorrhage 2 (CRASH-2), 64, 87
clot formation enhancement, 23
coagulopathy, 65–66, 95, 127
Combat Application Tourniquet (CAT), 13, 13*f*, 53, 54*f*
Combat Gauze, 24, 119
   directions, 24, 24*f*
Combat Ready Clamp (CRoC), 22, 23*f*, 54
Committee for Tactical Emergency Casualty Care (C-TECC), 1–2
Committee on Tactical Combat Casualty Care (Co-TCCC), 1, 2, 29, 46

communication
  evacuation care/cold zone
    patients, 95
    receiving hospitals, 96
  indirect threat care/warm zone
    patient, 79–80
    receiving hospitals, 80
compartment syndrome, 55
compensated shock, 58
complex airway device, 29
computed tomography (CT), 49
concealment, cover vs., 8, 9f
conduction, 70
CONTOMS program. See Counter
    Narcotics and Terrorism
    Operational Medical Support
    (CONTOMS) program
convection, 70
conversion of tourniquet
  evacuation care/cold zone
    contraindications for, 90, 126
    Plus-1, 88–90, 89f
    procedures, 88
  indirect threat care/warm zone, 22, 119
Co-TCCC. See Committee on Tactical
    Combat Casualty Care
Counter Narcotics and Terrorism
    Operational Medical Support
    (CONTOMS) program, 8
cover vs. concealment, 8, 9f
CPR. See cardiopulmonary resuscitation
CRASH-2. See Clinical Randomization of
    an Antifibrinolytic in Significant
    Hemorrhage 2
cricothyroid membrane, 32–33, 36, 120
cricothyrotomy, surgical, 31–32, 31f,
    111, 112f
  bougie-assisted placement of ET tube
    in surgical airway, 35, 35f, 36f
  incision, 33–34, 34f
  insert and secure endotracheal tube,
    34, 34f, 35f
  surface landmarks, 32–33, 32f, 33f, 34f
CRoC. See Combat Ready Clamp
C-TECC. See Committee for Tactical
    Emergency Casualty Care
Cushing's triad, 72
CYANOKIT, 92, 92f
cyanosis, 48b, 112b
Cyklokapron, 65

D

damage control resuscitation (DCR)
  coagulopathy and "lethal triad," 65–66
  TECC, 66
DCR. See damage control resuscitation
dead space, 41

Department of Defense (DoD), 66
diaphragm, 41
Difficult Airway Society, 32, 32f
direct pressure to wound, 20, 20f
direct threat care/hot zone, 3, 4f, 4t, 108
  constantly changing threat
    environment, 7–8
  cover vs. concealment, 8, 9f
  "get off the X," 7
  medical interventions in
    controlling massive hemorrhage,
      12–13
    placing patient in recovery position,
      12, 12f
    tourniquets, types of, 13–14, 13f, 14f
  mitigation of direct threats, 8
  operating in, 7
  primary medical priority in, 109,
    128–129
  rescue considerations
    drag and carry options, 10–12, 11f,
      12f, 14–15
    operational performance, 10
    rapid and remote assessment
      methodology, 8–10, 9f, 108–109
distal tibial insertion, 63f
distended neck veins, 48b, 112b,
    120–121
distributive (or vasogenic) shock, 57, 57t
documentation
  evacuation care/cold zone, 95–96,
    114–112
  indirect threat care/warm zone,
    74, 74f
drag and carry options, 109
  fore/aft carry, 12, 15
  one-person drag, 10–11, 11f, 14, 109f
  pack strap/Hawes carry, 11–12, 12f, 15
  two-person drag, 11, 11f, 14
  two-person side-by-side carry, 11,
    11f, 14

E

Emergency and Military Tourniquet,
    13, 13f, 53, 54f
Emergency Medical Resources Center
    (EMRC), 96
emergency surgical airway, 39
  steps, 33
emphysema, subcutaneous, 48b, 112b
EMRC. See Emergency Medical
    Resources Center
endotracheal (ET) tube
  bougie-assisted placement of, 35,
    35f, 36f
  inserting, 34, 34f
  securing, 35f

eschar, 78
evacuation care/cold zone, 3, 4f, 4t, 108,
    114–115, 125
  analgesia, 93, 94f
  breathing, 86–87, 87f
  burns, 91
    amyl nitrite, 92
    CYANOKIT, 92, 92f
    hydrogen cyanide poisoning
      protocol, 92–93
    sodium thiosulfate, 92
  cardiopulmonary resuscitation, 93–94
  hemorrhage control, 87–88
  hypothermia, 95, 95f
  indirect threat care/warm zone, 83
  needle decompression, 86–87, 87f
  primary, secondary, and tertiary
    evacuation plans, 84
  reassess, document, communicate, and
    prepare for movement, 95–96
  reassessment, 85
  shock management, 90
  situational awareness in, 83–84
  supraglottic airway, 85, 86f
  tourniquets
    contraindications for conversion, 90
    conversion procedures, 88
    Plus-1, 88–90, 89f
  tranexamic acid, 87–88
  transport resources, 84, 84f
  traumatic brain injury, 90–91
    altered mental status with, 90
    fluid resuscitation of, 91
evaporation, 70
explosives, 76, 76f
  breaches, 76
  robotic delivery of, 76
exsanguination, 12
external respiration, 43
extremity lift, 79, 79f
extremity tourniquets
  conversion contradictions, 22
  optimization, 21–22
  venous tourniquets, 22
EZ-IO, 62

F

face-to-face intubation, 31
Federal Emergency Management
    Agency (FEMA), 1
fentanyl, 79
fire and bombs as weapons, 75, 75f, 124
  explosives, 76, 76f
  public safety fire ignition sources, 76
fluid resuscitation
  of burned patients, 78, 78b
  of hemorrhagic shock, 60

for patients without traumatic brain injury, 90, 126
of traumatic brain injury, 91
fore/aft carry, 12, 15
fractures, pelvic, 56
full-thickness burns, 77–78, 78f

G

Glasgow Coma Scale (GCS), 71–72, 71f, 91, 123
good medicine and bad tactics, 5, 117
Grading of Recommendations Assessment, Development and Evaluation (GRADE), 93
gunshot wound, 44, 44f, 113f

H

Halo chest seal, 45, 45f
hemorrhage control
　assessing casualty for, 88, 125
　direct threat care/hot zone, 8, 12–13, 109
　evacuation care/cold zone, 87–88
　indirect threat care/warm zone, 56, 110–111, 111f. See also indirect threat care/warm zone
hemorrhagic shock, 21, 21t
　Class I hemorrhage, 58, 59f
　Class II hemorrhage, 58, 59f
　Class III hemorrhage, 58–59, 59f
　Class IV hemorrhage, 59–60, 60f
　classification of, 58–59, 59t
　fluid resuscitation of, 60, 61, 114, 122, 130
hemostatic dressings, 23–24
hydrogen cyanide poisoning protocol, 92–93
hydroxocobalamin, 92
hypercarbia, 91
hypertension, intracranial, 72
hypocarbia, 91
hypoglycemia, 91
hypotension, 66, 91, 123
hypothermia, 127
　evacuation care/cold zone, 95, 127
　　prevention and management kit, 95f
　indirect threat care/warm zone, 69
　　aspect of lethal triad, 70, 70f
　　preventing, 70–71
　　prevention and management kits, 71, 71f
hypoventilation, 43
hypovolemic shock, 57, 57t, 58, 121, 122
　decompensated, 61
　signs associated with, 61t
hypoxemia, 43
hypoxia, 43, 91

I

IEDS. See improvised explosive devices
immediate responders, importance of, 107
improvised explosive devices (IEDS), 22
improvised tourniquet, 14, 14f
incision, cricothyrotomy, 33–34, 34f
incremental exsanguination, 90
indirect threat care/warm zone, 3, 4f, 4t, 108
　airway in, 111–112. See also pediatric airways
　　adult vs. pediatric, 36, 36f, 37f
　　advanced pediatric airways, 38, 38f
　　emergency surgical airway, 39
　　nasopharyngeal airway, 28–29, 28f, 39
　　orotracheal and nasotracheal intubation, 31, 31f
　　recovery position, 29, 29f
　　sit-up/lean forward position, 29
　　supraglottic airways, 29–31, 30f, 39
　　surgical cricothyrotomy. See surgical cricothyrotomy
　　trauma jaw thrust and chin lift maneuvers, 27–28, 28f
　analgesia, 75
　burn care, 76–77
　　analgesia, 79
　　assessment of burn injury, 77–78, 77f, 78f
　　fluid resuscitation of burned patients, 78, 78b
　　smoke inhalation, fluid management considerations, 78–79
　circulation in. See circulation, indirect threat care/warm zone
　communication
　　with patient, 79–80
　　with receiving hospitals, 80
　CPR in multicasualty event, 80
　correct tension pneumothorax, 80
　evacuation care/cold zone and, 83–84, 84f
　fire and bombs as weapons, 75, 75f
　　explosives, 76, 76f
　　public safety fire ignition sources, 76
　hypothermia, 69
　　of lethal triad, 70, 70f
　　preventing, 70–71
　　prevention and management kits, 71, 71f
　ketamine, 75
　moving patients, 79, 79f, 80, 124
　patient assessment and massive hemorrhage interventions
　　assessment and intervention priorities, 18–19, 19f
　　asymmetrical response, 18, 18f
　　axillary hemorrhage, 25
　　bleeding assessment, 19, 19f
　　Combat Gauze directions, 24, 24f
　　direct pressure, 20, 20f
　　extremity tourniquets, 21–22
　　hemostatic dressings, 23–24
　　inguinal hemorrhage, 24–25
　　junctional hemorrhage. See junctional hemorrhage
　　progressive and aggressive intervention plan, 20, 20f
　　scene safety, 17–18
　　threat management, 18, 18f
　penetrating eye trauma, 79
　primary medical priority in, 110, 129
　reassess, monitor, and document patient, 72–73
　　documentation, 74, 74f
　　monitoring, 74
　　obtaining vital signs, 74
　　secondary survey, 73–74, 73f
　respiration/breathing
　　anatomy and physiology of, 41–43, 42f
　　chest seals, 46–47, 46f
　　needle decompression, 48–50, 49f
　　open pneumothorax, 44–45, 44f, 45f, 46f
　　oxygenation and ventilation process, 43
　　pathophysiology, 43
　　tension pneumothorax, 47–48, 47f
　traumatic brain injury assessment and intervention
　　Glasgow Coma Scale, 71–72, 71f
　　Cushing's triad, 72
　　intracranial hypertension, 72
　　intervention, 72
　triaging patients in, 80, 124
inguinal hemorrhage, 24–25
injury severity scores (ISS), 69
inspiration, negative pressure during, 41, 44
intact chest wall, 41, 44
internal (cellular) respiration, 43
interstitial space, 43
intracranial hypertension, 72
intraosseous access, 62–64, 62f, 63–64f, 66–67
intraosseous gun, 62f
intraosseous line, establishment of, 90
intraosseous needles, 62f
intrapulmonary pressure during ventilation phases, 42f
intravenous access, 62–64, 62f, 63–64f
intravenous (IV) line, establishment of, 90
intubating laryngeal mask airway, 30f
　with endotracheal tube in place, 30f

intubation, pediatric, 38
ischemia, organ tolerance to, 57t
ISS. See injury severity scores

J

Junctional Emergency Treatment Tool (JETT), 23, 23f, 56
junctional hemorrhage
  axillary, 25
  Combat Ready Clamp, 22, 23f
  inguinal, 24–25
  Junctional Emergency Treatment Tool, 23, 23f
  junctional tourniquets, 22
  SAM Junctional Tourniquet, 23, 23f
junctional tourniquets, 22, 111, 129

K

kaolin, 24
ketamine, 75, 114, 123, 130
King laryngotracheal airway, 30f

L

laryngeal handshake, 32, 32f
laryngeal mask airway (LMA), 30f
lethal triad, 65–66
  hypothermia aspect of, 70, 70f
LMA. See laryngeal mask airway
"look, listen, and feel" approach, 73
lung wounds, 44
Lysteda, 65

M

MARCH (Massive hemorrhage, Airway, Respiration, Circulation, and Head/Hypothermia) algorithm, 108, 128
  casualty response to, 104
  direct threat care/warm zone, 10
  evacuation care/cold zone, 83
  indirect threat care/warm zone, 18–19. See also indirect threat care/warm zone
mass-casualty event
  defined, 99
  emergency, 5
  scene safety, 17
mass-casualty incident (MCI), 1, 1f
medical intervention, direct threat care/hot zone, 8
  tourniquets, types of, 13–14, 13f, 14f
  placing patient in recovery position, 12, 12f
  controlling massive hemorrhage, 12–13
Military Application of Tranexamic Acid in Trauma Emergency and Resuscitation (MATTERs), 64–65

monitoring the patient, 74
morphine, 79
Mumbai terrorist attacks, 75, 75f

N

naloxone, 75, 114
narcotic medications, for pain, 75, 79, 114
nasopharyngeal airway (NPA), 28–29, 28f, 39, 119
  pediatric, 36–37
nasotracheal intubation, 31, 31f
National Highway Traffic Safety Administration, 93
National Joint Counterterrorism Awareness Workshop, 2
needle decompression (NDC), 3, 117
  evacuation care/cold zone, 86–87, 87f, 117
    needle/catheter size, 87, 125
  indirect threat care/warm zone, 48–49, 49f, 50–51
    assessing effectiveness of, 50
    bilateral for traumatic cardiac arrest, 50
    needle/catheter size, 50, 121
    pediatric tension pneumothorax, 50
    procedure, 49–50
    of thoracic cavity, 49f
neurogenic shock, 61–62, 122
  signs associated with, 61t
  vs. spinal shock, 61b
New Brunswick Trauma Program, 55, 56
NPA. See nasopharyngeal airway

O

on-scene situational assessment, 7
one-person drag, 10–11, 11f, 14, 109f
open pneumothorax, 113, 120
  assessment and management of, 44–45, 44f, 45f, 46f
  gunshot or stab wound, 44, 44f, 113f
operational performance, 10
orotracheal intubation, 31, 31f
oxycodone, 75, 114, 123, 130
oxygen, 42, 42f
  consumption, 43
  delivery, 43
  saturation via pulse oximetry, 91, 126
  tankers. See red blood cells
oxygenation, 43

P

PACE methodology. See Primary, Alternative, Contingency, Emergency (PACE) methodology
pack strap/Hawes carry, 11–12, 12f, 15

pediatrics
  airways
    adult vs., 36, 36f, 37f, 38, 120
    advanced airways, 38, 38f
    nasopharyngeal airway, 36–37
    supraglottic airways, 37–38
  tension pneumothorax, 50
palm method, for burns, 77, 77f
partial-thickness burns, 77, 77f
passive airway maintenance, 14, 118
patient movement, preparation for, 95–96
pelvic binders, 55–56, 56f
  application of, 56
  indications and contraindications for use, 56
  pelvic fractures stabilization, 56
  pelvic hemorrhage control, 56
penetrating eye trauma, 79
penetrating wound, 44. See also open pneumothorax
percutaneous needle cricothyrotomy, 38, 38f
PHTLS. See Prehospital Trauma Life Support
physical assessment of trauma patient, 73–74, 73f
Plus-1 tourniquet, 88–90, 89f
pneumatic tourniquet, 13
pneumothorax
  open. See open pneumothorax
  tension. See tension pneumothorax
positive-pressure ventilation, 47
Prehospital Trauma Life Support (PHTLS), 46, 113
primary brain injury, 71
primary triage, 100, 100f, 127
Primary, Alternative, Contingency, Emergency (PACE) methodology, 20, 119
  for evacuation planning, 84
progressive and aggressive intervention plan, 20, 20f
proximal tibial insertion, 63f
public safety fire ignition sources, 76
Pulse nightclub event, 17
Pyng FAST1, 62
pyrotechnic/incendiary tear gas, 76

R

radiation, 70
radio frequency identification (RFID) triage tags, 74, 95
raking, 19, 20, 87, 119, 125
rapid and remote assessment methodology (RAM), 8–10, 9f, 108–109
  key factor of, 12, 118

rapid four-step technique (RFST), 35
reassessing the patient
    evacuation care/cold zone, 85, 95–96
    indirect threat care/warm zone,
        72–74, 73*f*
recovery position
    direct threat care/hot zone, 12, 12*f*
    indirect threat care/warm zone, 29,
        29*f*, 111–112, 111*f*, 129
red blood cells (RBCs), 42–43
remote observation, 9
rescue task force (RTF), 5-6, 6*f*
residential structure targets, 76
respiration/breathing
    evacuation care/cold zone, 86–87, 87*f*
    indirect threat care/warm zone
        anatomy and physiology of
            breathing, 41–43, 42*f*
        chest seals, 46–47, 46*f*
        needle decompression, 48–50, 49*f*
        open pneumothorax, 44–45, 44*f*,
            45*f*, 46*f*
        oxygenation and ventilation
            process, 43
        pathophysiology, 43
        sounds decreasing on injured side,
            48*b*, 112*b*
        tension pneumothorax, 47–48, 47*f*
restoration of spontaneous circulation
    (ROSC), 93
resuscitation zones. *See specific zones*
RFST. *See* rapid four-step technique
Ringer solution, 60
robotic delivery of explosives, 76
RTF. *See* rescue task force

S

Sacco triage method (STM), 103
SALT triage. *See* Sort, Assess, Lifesaving
        interventions, and Treatment
        and/or Transport (SALT) triage
SAM chest seal, 45, 45*f*
SAM Junctional Tourniquet (SJT), 23,
    23*f*, 56
scene safety, 17–18
school bombing targets, 76
secondary survey, 73–74, 73*f*
    penetrating eye trauma, 79, 124
secondary triage decisions, 104*f*
    casualty response to MARCH
        treatments, 104
    tactical situation, 103–104
"Sharpie" style permanent marker, 74
shock
    defined, 56, 57, 121
    evacuation care/cold zone, 90
    hemorrhagic, 21, 21*t*

indirect threat care/warm zone, 114
    assessment, 56–57, 57*t*
    fluid resuscitation of hemorrhagic
        shock, 60
    hemorrhagic, 58–60, 58*f*, 59*f*, 59*t*, 60*f*
    hypovolemic, 57*t*, 58
    neurogenic, 61–62
    signs associated with types, 61*t*
    types of traumatic, 57*t*
Simple Triage And Rapid Treatment
    (START) triage, 101, 102*f*
situational awareness in evacuation
    care/cold zone, 83–84
situations, tactical care
    direct threat care/hot zone, 3, 4*f*, 4*t*
    evacuation care/cold zone, 3, 4*f*, 4*t*
    indirect threat care/warm zone, 3, 4*f*, 4*t*
sit-up/lean forward position, in indirect
    threat care/warm zone, 29
SJT. *See* SAM Junctional Tourniquet
smoke inhalation, 77, 78–79, 91, 93, 126
sodium nitrite, 93
sodium thiosulfate, 92, 93
SOFTT. *See* Special Operations Forces
    Tactical Tourniquet
SOFTT Gen 4, 13
SOFTT Wide, 13
Sort, Assess, Lifesaving interventions,
    and Treatment and/or Transport
    (SALT) triage, 101–103,
    103*f*, 128
Special Operations Forces Tactical
    Tourniquet (SOFTT), 13, 13*f*,
    53, 54*f*
special weapons and tactics (SWAT)
    teams, 9, 107
spinal shock, neurogenic shock *vs.*, 61*b*
stab wound, 44, 44*f*, 113*f*
START triage. *See* Simple Triage And
    Rapid Treatment (START) triage
sternal insertion, 63*f*
STM. *See* Sacco triage method
stun/flash bang grenade, 76
subcutaneous emphysema, 48*b*, 112*b*
sucking chest wound, 44
supraglottic airway
    evacuation care/cold zone, 85,
        86*f*, 125
    indirect threat care/warm zone, 29–31,
        30*f*, 39
    pediatric, 37–38
surface landmarks, of cricothyrotomy,
    32–33, 32*f*, 33*f*, 34*f*
sweep-and-rake assessment, 19, 87
sweeping, 19, 87
sympathetic nervous system, 58,
    60, 122

T

tachycardia, 58
Tactical Emergency Casualty Care (TECC)
    caregivers' first responsibility, 108, 128
    course
        coming from, 1–2
        goals of, 4–5
        information sources of, 2
        offering skill stations, 2–3
        16-hour classroom course
            covering, 2
    damage control resuscitation, 66
    description of, 1
    guiding principles, 4–5
    mass-casualty management, 1*f*
    other elements operating within
        tactical environment
        rescue task force, 5–6, 6*f*
        tactical emergency medical
            support, 6
    phases of, 2, 108. *See also specific phases*
    response and arrival-scene
        assessment, 5
    tactical care situations
        direct threat care/hot zone, 3, 4*f*, 4*t*
        evacuation care/cold zone, 3, 4*f*, 4*t*
        indirect threat care/warm zone,
            3, 4*f*, 4*t*
tactical emergency medical support
    (TEMS), 6
target compression devices (TCDs), 23
TECC. *See* Tactical Emergency Casualty
    Care
TEMS. *See* tactical emergency medical
    support
tension pneumothorax, 3, 47–48, 47*f*,
    112, 117
    correct, 80
    pediatric, 50
    signs of, 48*b*, 112*b*, 113, 120–121, 130
Terrorism and Political Violence, 84
thermal imaging technology, 9
ThinkSharp Inc., 103
thoracic cavity, needle decompression of,
    49*f*, 87*f*
thoracic injury, 47
threat environment, constantly
    changing, 7–8
threat management, 18, 18*f*
time-sensitive prehospital treatments,
    96, 115, 127, 130
tourniquets, 110–111. *See also specific
    types*
    application, 15, 54–55, 54*f*, 55*b*
    arterial, 55
    assessment, 53–54, 54*f*
    Combat Application, 13, 13*f*

Index   **135**

tourniquets (*Continued*)
  Emergency and Military, 13, 13*f*
  extremity. *See* extremity tourniquets
  improvised, 14, 14*f*
  insufficient compression, 55, 121
  Special Operations Forces Tactical, 13, 13*f*
  time limit, 55
tracheal deviation, 48*b*, 112*b*
tracheal hook, 35, 35*f*
tranexamic acid (TXA)
  evacuation care/cold zone, 87–88
  indirect threat care/warm zone, 64–65, 111, 129
    administration, 65, 67, 123
transport resources, for evacuation care, 84, 84*f*
trauma chin lift maneuver, 27–28, 28*f*
trauma jaw thrust maneuver, 27–28, 28*f*
traumatic brain injury (TBI), 66, 123
  assessment
    Cushing's triad, 72
    Glasgow Coma Scale, 71–72, 71*f*
    intracranial hypertension, 72

evacuation care/cold zone, 90–91
  altered mental status with, 90
  fluid resuscitation of, 91
intervention, 72
traumatic cardiac arrest (TCA), 80, 93
  bilateral needle decompression for, 50
  causes in evacuation care/cold zone, 94, 126
triage
  concepts, 99–100
  critique of, 101, 127
  indirect threat care/warm zone, 74, 74*f*
  limitations of, 100–101
  primary, 100, 100*f*
  Sacco triage method, 103
  SALT triage, 101–103, 103*f*
  secondary triage decisions, 104*f*
    casualty response to MARCH treatments, 104
    tactical situation, 103–104
  START triage, 101, 102*f*
  tags, 95, 95*f*, 115, 115*f*

two-person drag, 11, 11*f*, 14
two-person side-by-side carry, 11, 11*f*, 14
Tylenol. *See* acetaminophen

U
underlying lung, injury to, 45, 120
U.S. Bomb Data Center (USBDC), 76

V
venous tourniquets, 22
vented chest seals, 46, 46*f*
ventilation, 43
  positive-pressure, 47
vital signs, obtaining, 74

W
weapons
  and communications equipment, securing, 18, 18*f*
  fire and bombs as, 75, 75*f*, 124
    explosives, 76, 76*f*
    public safety fire ignition sources, 76